Soft Tissue and Musculoskeletal Medicine in Rheumatology

AF871910

Raj Amarnani

Soft Tissue and Musculoskeletal Medicine in Rheumatology

Springer

Raj Amarnani
Consultant in Sport, Exercise & Musculoskeletal Medicine
University College London Hospitals NHS Foundation Trust
London, UK

ISBN 978-3-032-29440-1 ISBN 978-3-032-29441-8 (eBook)
https://doi.org/10.1007/978-3-032-29441-8

© The Editor(s) (if applicable) and The Author(s), under exclusive license to Springer Nature Switzerland AG 2026

This work is subject to copyright. All rights are solely and exclusively licensed by the Publisher, whether the whole or part of the material is concerned, specifically the rights of translation, reprinting, reuse of illustrations, recitation, broadcasting, reproduction on microfilms or in any other physical way, and transmission or information storage and retrieval, electronic adaptation, computer software, or by similar or dissimilar methodology now known or hereafter developed.
The use of general descriptive names, registered names, trademarks, service marks, etc. in this publication does not imply, even in the absence of a specific statement, that such names are exempt from the relevant protective laws and regulations and therefore free for general use.
The publisher, the authors and the editors are safe to assume that the advice and information in this book are believed to be true and accurate at the date of publication. Neither the publisher nor the authors or the editors give a warranty, expressed or implied, with respect to the material contained herein or for any errors or omissions that may have been made. The publisher remains neutral with regard to jurisdictional claims in published maps and institutional affiliations.

This Springer imprint is published by the registered company Springer Nature Switzerland AG
The registered company address is: Gewerbestrasse 11, 6330 Cham, Switzerland

If disposing of this product, please recycle the paper.

This book is dedicated to my family—Dad, Mum, Manini, Kunal and Meenakshi—whose unwavering support has underpinned every stage of my career. Your belief in me, through the ups and downs of my health, training and clinical work, has made everything that followed possible. Thank you for always giving me the confidence to keep going.

Preface

This book was shaped by a gap I have continued to encounter in clinical practice: the widening space between rheumatology and soft tissue musculoskeletal medicine.

Rheumatology has historically been rooted in the assessment of musculoskeletal pain and function. In recent years, the specialty has quite rightly made enormous advances in immunology and the treatment of inflammatory disease. However, the reality of day-to-day clinical practice is often less clear-cut. Patients rarely present in defined categories. Instead, they present with overlapping features: tendon pain, enthesopathy and regional syndromes that sit at the interface of mechanical load, inflammation and systemic disease.

Through my work across rheumatology, sport and exercise medicine and elite sporting environments, I have seen how frequently these problems are either under-recognised or managed in isolation. This can lead to delayed diagnoses, fragmented care and suboptimal outcomes.

There is a tendency to separate "inflammatory" from "mechanical" pathology. In practice, this distinction is often artificial. Many of the most challenging cases lie precisely in that overlap.

The aim of this book is to provide a practical, clinically grounded framework for approaching soft tissue presentations within a rheumatological context. The emphasis is on how to think, not just what to know-on clinical reasoning, pattern recognition and decision-making in real-world settings.

Rehabilitation and function sit at the centre of this approach. Imaging and interventions have an important role, but they are rarely the solution in isolation. The focus throughout is on integrating these elements to support meaningful patient outcomes.

This book reflects how I approach musculoskeletal medicine in practice: combining principles from rheumatology, sport and exercise medicine and rehabilitation to deliver care that is both precise and pragmatic.

London, UK

Raj Amarnani

Acknowledgements

I have been fortunate to train and work alongside outstanding clinicians across rheumatology, sport and exercise medicine and rehabilitation. Their expertise, insight and willingness to challenge my thinking have been instrumental in shaping my clinical approach.

I am particularly grateful to the multidisciplinary teams I have worked with: physiotherapists, orthopaedic surgeons, radiologists, pharmacists, occupational therapists, nurses and fellow physicians, whose collaborative approach continues to influence how I manage complex musculoskeletal presentations.

I would also like to thank the patients I have cared for. Their experiences, resilience and trust have been central to the development of the perspectives shared in this book.

Finally, thank you to my family for their continued support throughout my training and career.

Competing Interests The author has no competing interests to declare that are relevant to the content of this manuscript.

About the Book

This textbook provides a clinically focused approach to soft tissue and musculoskeletal conditions encountered in rheumatology.

It brings together principles from rheumatology, sport and exercise medicine and rehabilitation to address a group of conditions that are common, often complex and frequently underrepresented in traditional rheumatology texts.

Structured by anatomical region, the book covers key soft-tissue presentations including tendinopathies, enthesopathies, bursitis and regional pain syndromes. It also explores how these conditions intersect with inflammatory disease and how to approach this overlap with clarity and confidence.

A central theme throughout is the integration of diagnosis and management—moving beyond isolated labels towards a more functional and patient-centred model of care.

Key features include:

- A structured approach to clinical assessment and diagnostic reasoning
- Practical guidance on the use of imaging and investigations
- Region-specific management strategies grounded in real-world practice
- Integration of rehabilitation and exercise-based principles
- Thoughtful use of interventions, including ultrasound-guided procedures

This book is written for rheumatologists, sport and exercise medicine physicians, physiotherapists and other clinicians involved in musculoskeletal care who want a clearer, more integrated approach to soft tissue pathology.

Contents

About the Author

Raj Amarnani is a Consultant in Sport, Exercise and Musculoskeletal Medicine at University College London Hospitals NHS Foundation Trust, based in London, United Kingdom. His clinical work spans NHS and elite sport environments, with a specialist focus on complex musculoskeletal presentations, soft tissue disorders, diagnostic ultrasound, ultrasound-guided interventions, bone health and the interface between rheumatology and musculoskeletal medicine.

He is President of the Rheumatology and Rehabilitation Section at the Royal Society of Medicine, Chair of the British Society for Rheumatology Physical Activity Specialist Interest Group, and a trustee and medical advisor to the National Axial Spondyloarthritis Society. He also contributes to international guideline development through European Alliance of Associations for Rheumatology taskforces, including work on physical activity and fatigue in rheumatic and musculoskeletal diseases.

Dr Amarnani completed his medical degree with distinction, receiving multiple academic prizes during his training, before undertaking an MSc in Musculoskeletal Sciences at the University of Oxford. He holds Membership of the Royal College of Physicians and Fellowship of the Faculty of Sport and Exercise Medicine. His academic work includes more than 100 peer-reviewed publications in leading journals, including *The Lancet Rheumatology* and the *British Journal of Sports Medicine*, with a focus on musculoskeletal medicine, rheumatic disease and the role of physical activity in long-term conditions.

Alongside his clinical and academic work, Dr Amarnani has extensive experience in elite sport, supporting athletes across cricket, football, basketball, tennis and dance as well as working with national and international teams and at major sporting events. This has given him a broad perspective on soft tissue injury, load-related pain, rehabilitation and return to activity, which complements his work in rheumatology and long-term musculoskeletal conditions.

Through this combination of physician training, specialist musculoskeletal expertise, rheumatology leadership, academic research and elite sport experience, Dr Amarnani is uniquely placed to write a practical guide to soft tissue and musculoskeletal medicine in rheumatology. His work bridges specialties that are often considered separately, helping clinicians approach non-articular and soft tissue presentations with greater confidence, precision and clinical reasoning.

Introduction: Scope of Soft Tissue Rheumatology

1

Abstract

Musculoskeletal *soft tissue rheumatology* encompasses a broad spectrum of non-articular conditions affecting tendons, ligaments, bursae, fascia and related structures. These disorders, often termed *soft tissue rheumatism*, are extremely common and impose a substantial burden on patients and healthcare systems. In fact, soft tissue pain syndromes like back pain, neck pain and shoulder pain rank among the most prevalent medical complaints worldwide (Natvig and Picavet, Best Pract Res Clin Rheumatol. 16:777–93, 2002). This chapter outlines the scope and importance of soft tissue rheumatology, defines key concepts (such as tendinopathy, bursitis, enthesopathy, etc.) and previews the case-based approach used throughout this book. A brief clinical scenario will illustrate the challenge of distinguishing soft tissue pain from inflammatory joint disease, setting the stage for the detailed regional chapters to follow.

Prevalence and Impact of Soft Tissue Musculoskeletal Conditions

Soft tissue rheumatic conditions are far more common than many classic inflammatory rheumatic diseases. Epidemiologic studies show a high point prevalence of regional musculoskeletal pain in the general population—for example, neck pain in about 10–19% of adults, shoulder pain in 18–26%, elbow pain in 8–12% and wrist/hand pain in roughly 9–17% [1]. Low back pain is particularly widespread: in 2020, an estimated 619 million people globally had low back pain, and it is *the single leading cause of disability worldwide* [2]. Almost all of us will experience back or neck pain at least once in their life. The lifetime prevalence of back pain approaches 60–80% and for neck pain ranges around 20–70% in various studies [1]. These soft tissue conditions collectively represent a major public health issue with huge economic costs due to healthcare utilisation and lost work productivity [2].

© The Author(s), under exclusive license to Springer Nature Switzerland AG 2026

R. Amarnani, *Soft Tissue and Musculoskeletal Medicine in Rheumatology*,
https://doi.org/10.1007/978-3-032-29441-8_1

Soft tissue rheumatism is *defined as clinical conditions arising from structures around joints—tendons, bursae, ligaments, fascia and muscles* [3]. Because these nonarticular pains are so ubiquitous, they account for a large proportion of musculoskeletal complaints seen by physicians. Indeed, *the most common reason for a rheumatology consult is musculoskeletal pain*, which must first be sorted into articular (joint) vs nonarticular (soft tissue) sources. In primary care, many patients with shoulder, back or knee pain ultimately have soft tissue aetiologies rather than an inflammatory condition. Rheumatologists often encounter the more severe or refractory cases of soft tissue rheumatism, but mild to moderate cases are managed daily by general medicine physicians, orthopaedic surgeons, sports medicine physicians and physiotherapists.

Despite their high frequency, soft tissue rheumatic disorders have sometimes been underrecognised or misunderstood. Unlike well-defined diseases such as rheumatoid arthritis with clear diagnostic criteria, many soft tissue pain syndromes lack universally accepted definitions and specific diagnostic tests. Terms like "regional pain syndrome" or "soft tissue rheumatism" encompass a heterogeneous group of conditions. Patients may simply report "joint pain" or "muscle pain," which requires careful clinical evaluation to pinpoint a soft tissue cause. Nonetheless, the *impact of these conditions on society is enormous*, contributing to chronic pain, disability and healthcare costs [4]. For example, chronic widespread pain (including fibromyalgia) affects an estimated 10–15% of adults globally, and fibromyalgia syndrome itself—characterised by diffuse soft tissue pain and tenderness, occurs in roughly 2% of the population [3]. By sheer numbers, soft tissue rheumatic ailments (back pain, neck/shoulder syndromes, tendon injuries, etc.) far outnumber inflammatory arthritides like rheumatoid arthritis (which has around 0.5–1% prevalence). Thus, having a solid grasp of soft tissue rheumatology is crucial for clinicians in rheumatology and primary care alike.

Key Concepts and Definitions

Soft tissue rheumatology comprises a variety of specific conditions. Before delving into regional syndromes, it is important to understand some key terms and concepts:

- *Tendinopathy:* This is a broad term referring to *any disorder of a tendon* that causes pain or impaired function. It includes both *tendinitis* and *tendinosis*. *Tendinitis* refers to *acute inflammation of a tendon* (often from microtears due to overload) [5]. Tendinitis is the classic "tendonitis" scenario of a tendon acutely irritated by injury or overuse, causing pain, tenderness and sometimes swelling. If the tendon injury fails to heal and inflammation becomes chronic, degenerative changes can ensue. *Tendinosis* describes *chronic degeneration of tendon collagen fibres*, with disorganised structure and little active inflammation [5]. Tendinosis tends to develop from repetitive strain or aging, leading to a weak, thickened tendon. In practice, many persistent tendon pains (like chronic tennis elbow or Achilles tendon pain) are tendinoses. Because inflammation and degeneration often overlap, clinicians use *tendinopathy* as an umbrella term encompassing both acute inflammatory tendon injuries and chronic degenerative tendon conditions [5]. Common examples include rotator cuff tendinopathy, lateral epicondylitis (tennis elbow) and patellar tendinopathy.

- *Bursitis:* A bursa is a small fluid-filled sac that cushions and reduces friction between moving tissues (e.g. between a tendon and bone). *Bursitis* means *inflammation of a bursa*, usually resulting in swelling, pain and tenderness around a joint. Bursae are found around most major joints; when they become irritated from overuse, trauma or other causes, they can fill with excess fluid. *Bursitis is a painful inflammation of the bursae that cushion bones, tendons and muscles near joints* [6]. Common sites include the subacromial bursa in the shoulder (subacromial bursitis), the olecranon bursa at the elbow (olecranon bursitis), prepatellar bursa in the knee (housemaid's knee) and trochanteric bursae at the lateral hip (trochanteric bursitis). Clinically, bursitis often presents with localised swelling and pain that is exacerbated by movements compressing the bursa. It can sometimes be difficult to distinguish from arthritis of the joint, but bursitis typically causes extraarticular swelling and point tenderness over the bursal sac rather than true joint line pain.
- *Enthesopathy:* An enthesis is the site where a tendon, ligament or joint capsule attaches to the bone. *Enthesopathy* refers to *any disorder of these attachment sites (entheses)*, often involving degenerative or inflammatory changes. In simple terms, enthesopathy is "something wrong with the enthesis"—the connective tissue insertion point [7]. This broad term includes both mechanical enthesopathies (due to repetitive stress or overuse at the tendon insertion) and inflammatory enthesitis related to autoimmune diseases. For example, chronic stress on the Achilles tendon insertion at the heel can lead to a degenerative enthesopathy (with calcification or spur formation), whereas in psoriatic arthritis or axial spondyloarthritis, you might see inflammatory *enthesitis* at the Achilles insertion. It is useful to distinguish *enthesitis*, which specifically means *inflammation of an enthesis*, as a subset of enthesopathy [7]. Enthesitis is a hallmark of the seronegative *spondyloarthropathies*—patients with these conditions often have chronic heel pain, tibial tuberosity pain or other tendon insertion pain due to inflammation at the entheses. In contrast, purely mechanical enthesopathies result from overuse and are not driven by systemic inflammation. Both types present as localised tenderness at tendon insertions, and imaging (like ultrasound or MRI) may show thickening or calcifications at the enthesis.
- *Tenosynovitis:* Tendons that run through narrow channels or fibroosseous tunnels (such as those in the wrist and hand) are surrounded by a *tendon sheath* lined with synovial fluid. *Tenosynovitis* is *inflammation of a tendon sheath*—essentially an inflammatory process involving the synovial lining around a tendon [5]. This often occurs in the hand and wrist flexor tendons or in the tendons around the ankle. A well-known example is *De Quervain's tenosynovitis*, which affects the sheath of the thumb extensor tendons at the wrist, causing pain on thumb movement and a positive Finkelstein's test (pain with ulnar deviation of the wrist). Another example is *trigger finger*, caused by flexor tenosynovitis in a

finger—the inflamed tendon nodule catches at the pulley, causing the finger to lock or catch. Tenosynovitis can result from overuse, inflammatory diseases or occasionally infection. It often presents with tendon pain exacerbated by movement and sometimes palpable crepitus (a grating sensation) as the inflamed tendon sheath moves.

- *Other Terms: Soft tissue rheumatism* as a whole cover numerous conditions. Some are localised while others are more generalised. *Myofascial pain syndrome* refers to pain arising from muscle and its fascial attachments, often associated with trigger points (discrete tender knots within muscle that refer pain to distant areas). *Fibromyalgia*, discussed in Chap. 11, is a chronic widespread pain condition without overt tissue inflammation, believed to stem from central pain processing abnormalities—it can be considered a generalised soft tissue pain syndrome. Additionally, nerve compression or *entrapment syndromes* (such as carpal tunnel syndrome at the wrist or cubital tunnel syndrome at the elbow) are often included in the domain of soft tissue rheumatology because they cause musculoskeletal pain and are managed by similar nonsurgical approaches initially. This book will cover many of these terms and conditions in detail, but the above definitions provide a foundation.

By understanding these core concepts—tendinopathy, bursitis, enthesopathy/enthesitis, tenosynovitis, etc.—the reader will be equipped to parse the diagnoses discussed in later chapters.

A Case-Based Approach to Learning

Throughout this book, each chapter begins with a *clinical case vignette* that typifies the soft tissue condition under discussion. This case-based approach is used to ground the discussion in real-world scenarios and to engage the reader in clinical reasoning. Rather than presenting soft tissue rheumatology in the abstract, we illustrate each condition through the story of a patient—describing their symptoms, physical exam findings, diagnostic workup and management. This mirrors the way clinicians encounter these problems in practice. Case vignettes help highlight critical decision points, such as distinguishing between similar diagnoses or choosing an appropriate treatment plan.

For example, in the shoulder pain chapter (Chap. 4), we meet a middle-aged patient with chronic shoulder aching and use that case to explore the differential diagnosis of shoulder soft tissue disorders (rotator cuff tendinopathy, subacromial bursitis, adhesive capsulitis) vs other possibilities like glenohumeral arthritis. In the elbow chapter, a case of lateral elbow pain in a manual worker leads us through the recognition of tennis elbow and how to manage it with conservative measures. Each case is followed by an analysis of the clinical evaluation, relevant investigations (imaging or blood tests if needed) and evidence-based treatment options. This format allows the reader to "walk through" the diagnostic process and management decision-making as if in a clinical encounter. By the end of each chapter, the case is resolved with a management plan, and key learning points are summarised.

This case-driven approach underscores the importance of an individualised assessment. Two patients with seemingly similar complaints (e.g. knee pain) may have very different underlying causes—one might have patellar tendinopathy from overuse, while another has early rheumatoid arthritis affecting the knee joint. The case discussions emphasise how the history, physical exam and judicious use of imaging or tests can lead to the correct diagnosis, ensuring the patient receives appropriate therapy. A recurring theme will be the differentiation of *mechanical vs inflammatory pain*, which we will now introduce as one of the core challenges in rheumatology.

Differentiating Soft Tissue Versus Inflammatory Pain: A Diagnostic Challenge

One of the first tasks when evaluating any musculoskeletal complaint is to determine whether the pain is due to a *mechanical soft tissue issue* or an *inflammatory arthritic process*. Soft tissue rheumatic pains are generally *mechanical or degenerative* in nature—arising from overuse, wear-and-tear or minor injuries to tendons, bursae and related structures. In contrast, *inflammatory rheumatic diseases* often cause pain due to synovitis or systemic inflammation, often accompanied by heat, swelling, morning stiffness and other systemic features. Distinguishing between these broad categories is crucial, as it guides further workup and treatment. Mechanical soft tissue conditions are typically managed with activity modification, physiotherapy, local measures and analgesics, whereas inflammatory conditions may require immunomodulatory medications (e.g. corticosteroids, DMARDs (disease-modifying antirheumatic drugs) or biologics) and a different follow-up strategy.

There are several *key clinical differences* that can help differentiate inflammatory vs mechanical soft tissue pain:

- *Onset and duration:* Inflammatory arthritis often has an insidious onset in younger to mid-adult ages (e.g. inflammatory back pain from axial spondyloarthritis usually begins before 40). The pain tends to be chronic (>3 months). Mechanical pains can occur at any age and often follow an identifiable overuse or injury; acute mechanical pain is common, though chronic degenerative tendon or joint issues also occur in older adults.
- *Diurnal pattern (morning stiffness):* Prolonged *morning stiffness* is a hallmark of inflammatory conditions. Patients with inflammatory pain often wake up with significant stiffness and pain in the affected area, lasting *30 minutes or more* each morning or after periods of rest [8]. In *mechanical* soft tissue pain, there may be some morning discomfort, but it is typically mild (<15–20 minutes) and the patient "loosens up" quickly. Mechanical pain tends to worsen towards the end of an active day rather than primarily in the morning.

- *Effect of activity vs rest: Inflammatory pain* tends to *improve with moderate activity* and worsen after prolonged rest. Patients often report that moving around or doing light exercise eases their stiffness and pain (hence the classic description that inflammatory back pain improves with exercise) [8]. In contrast, *mechanical pain* usually *worsens with activity* and improves with rest. For example, a patient with rotator cuff tendinopathy will feel more shoulder pain after a day of heavy lifting, and relief when they rest the arm, whereas a patient with polymyalgia rheumatica feels worst upon waking and gets better after moving their shoulders.
- *Swelling and objective inflammation:* Inflammatory conditions often cause visible or palpable *swelling*, warmth and joint effusion (if a joint is involved) or diffuse tenderness at entheses. Soft tissue rheumatic conditions can cause local tenderness and sometimes mild swelling (e.g. a bulge over a bursitis or thickening of a tendon) but usually lack the pronounced joint swelling or *redness* seen in arthritis. For instance, in knee pain, a patellar tendinopathy might cause localised swelling at the front of the knee, but an *inflammatory arthritis of the knee* would cause a generalised joint effusion, warmth and reduced range of motion of the entire joint. Soft tissue issues typically do not cause *red, hot joints* (unless there is an acute trauma or infection).
- *Systemic symptoms: Constitutional symptoms* (fever, fatigue, weight loss) and laboratory evidence of inflammation (elevated ESR/CRP) are often present in systemic inflammatory rheumatic diseases but are absent in purely mechanical soft tissue problems. A patient with fibromyalgia or tennis elbow generally feels otherwise well aside from pain, whereas a patient with rheumatoid arthritis might have fatigue and elevated inflammatory markers along with joint pain. (Fibromyalgia is somewhat an exception in that it is noninflammatory but can coexist with fatigue and sleep disturbances, though without objective inflammation or lab abnormalities.)
- *Response to NSAIDs (nonsteroidal antiinflammatory drugs):* While not absolute, a dramatic response to NSAID medication is commonly reported in inflammatory arthritis (especially axial spondyloarthritis—inflammatory back pain often improves markedly with NSAIDs) [9]. Mechanical pains can also respond to NSAIDs for symptom relief, but the effect may be less pronounced. This observation can be a clue but should be interpreted with caution.

In practice, taking a thorough history and performing a focused physical exam are the most important tools to distinguish these causes. After identifying musculoskeletal pain, *it is important to determine if it is articular or nonarticular* and then tease out key features pointing to specific diagnoses. For example, consider *shoulder pain*: pain originating from rotator cuff tendons or subacromial bursa often hurts with active motion (especially overhead) but the shoulder's passive range of motion may be near normal, and there is localised tenderness over the greater tuberosity or subacromial area. In contrast, shoulder pain from *glenohumeral joint arthritis* (inflammatory or osteoarthritis) typically causes limitations in both active *and* passive range of motion, diffuse deep joint pain and possibly swelling of the joint capsule; also, arthritis pain often correlates with morning stiffness elsewhere or laboratory inflammation.

Case Scenario: Soft Tissue or Inflammatory?

Mrs. A is a 52-year-old avid gardener who presents with 3 months of right shoulder pain. She reports an achy pain around the lateral shoulder that began gradually, without any single injury. It hurts the most when she reaches overhead or tries to lift objects, and she has had to stop her weekly tennis games due to the pain. At times, the pain radiates down the upper arm. She notices some stiffness after her evening gardening, but in the mornings, her shoulder mainly feels a bit sore for only 5–10 minutes after getting out of bed. Rest provides relief, whereas activities like trimming hedges or painting aggravate the pain. She denies fevers, weight loss or other joint pains. On exam, Mrs. A has tenderness over the subacromial area and pain when abducting her arm between 60° and 120° (a positive "painful arc"). Her passive range of motion is nearly full (just mild pain at end range), but active motion is painful. There is no visible swelling of the shoulder joint and no warmth.

This scenario highlights the thought process in differentiating a soft tissue condition from an inflammatory one. Mrs. A's history of *activity-related worsening and relief with rest*, very minimal morning stiffness and lack of systemic symptoms point towards a *mechanical soft tissue aetiology*. The exam findings of a painful arc of motion and point tenderness over the rotator cuff region are classic for *rotator cuff tendinopathy or subacromial bursitis*, rather than an inflammatory arthritis. If this were an early inflammatory condition (like rheumatoid arthritis in the shoulder or polymyalgia rheumatica), one might expect more pronounced morning stiffness (e.g. difficulty raising arms for >30 minutes after waking), pain at rest/night, perhaps swelling or warmth in the joint and often involvement of other joints or constitutional symptoms. None of those are prominent here. Thus, the clinical picture strongly suggests a soft tissue rheumatism diagnosis (rotator cuff syndrome). Imaging, such as shoulder ultrasound or MRI, could be used to confirm a tendon tear or bursitis if needed, and treatment would focus on physiotherapy, activity modification and possibly a subacromial corticosteroid injection—quite different from the systemic medications, we would use for an inflammatory polyarthritis.

This case underscores the importance of careful clinical evaluation. Throughout the upcoming chapters, we will encounter similar scenarios in each anatomical region. By analysing the *history*, *physical exam* and appropriate use of *diagnostic tools* (imaging, blood tests), the clinician can usually distinguish soft tissue rheumatic conditions from articular or systemic ones. Chapters 2 and 3 will arm the reader with general approaches to history-taking, examination techniques and diagnostic investigations for musculoskeletal complaints. Then, Chaps. 4, 5, 6, 7, 8, 9, and 10 delve into specific regions (shoulder, elbow, hand/wrist, spine, hip, knee, foot/ankle) with prototypical cases and conditions. Chap. 11 addresses generalised soft tissue pain syndromes like fibromyalgia, and Chap. 12 integrates management principles across all these conditions.

In summary, *soft tissue rheumatology is a vital part of musculoskeletal medicine*, given the high prevalence and impact of tendon, bursal, enthesis and myofascial pain disorders. These conditions, while nonlife-threatening, cause significant pain and disability but are often very treatable once correctly diagnosed. Mastering the recognition of common entities—and differentiating them from inflammatory or other causes—is a key objective of this text. The case-based, thorough approach in this book aims to provide a *practical framework* for evaluating any patient with musculoskeletal pain, ensuring that diagnoses like "tendinopathy" or "bursitis" are made accurately and managed effectively. The next chapter will begin that journey by reviewing the fundamentals of *clinical evaluation* for soft tissue complaints, including history, physical examination manoeuvres and red flags not to miss.

References

1. Walker-Bone KE, Palmer KT, Reading I, Cooper C. Soft-tissue rheumatic disorders of the neck and upper limb: prevalence and risk factors. Semin Arthritis Rheum [Internet]. 2003;33(3):185–203. Available from: http://www.ncbi.nlm.nih.gov/pubmed/14671728
2. Zhang C, Lv B, Yi Q, Qiu G, Wu F. Global, regional, and national burden of low back pain in working-age population from 1990 to 2021 and projections for 2050. Front public Heal [Internet]. 2025;13:1559355. Available from: http://www.ncbi.nlm.nih.gov/pubmed/40342503
3. Dizner-Golab A, Lisowska B, Kosson D. Fibromyalgia - etiology, diagnosis and treatment including perioperative management in patients with fibromyalgia. Reumatologia [Internet]. 2023;61(2):137–48. Available from: http://www.ncbi.nlm.nih.gov/pubmed/37223370
4. Natvig B, Picavet HSJ. The epidemiology of soft tissue rheumatism. Best Pract Res Clin Rheumatol [Internet]. 2002;16(5):777–93. Available from: http://www.ncbi.nlm.nih.gov/pubmed/12473273
5. Millar NL, Silbernagel KG, Thorborg K, Kirwan PD, Galatz LM, Abrams GD, et al. Tendinopathy. Nat Rev Dis Prim [Internet]. 2021;7(1):1. Available from: https://www.nature.com/articles/s41572-020-00234-1
6. Aaron DL, Patel A, Kayiaros S, Calfee R. Four common types of bursitis: diagnosis and management. J Am Acad Orthop Surg [Internet]. 2011;19(6):359–67. Available from: http://www.ncbi.nlm.nih.gov/pubmed/21628647
7. Sudoł-Szopińska I, Kwiatkowska B, Prochorec-Sobieszek M, Maśliński W. Enthesopathies and enthesitis. Part 1. Etiopathogenesis. J Ultrason [Internet]. 2015;15(60):72–84. Available from: http://www.ncbi.nlm.nih.gov/pubmed/26674568
8. Poudel P, Lappin SL. Inflammatory arthritis [Internet]. In: StatPearls; 2026. Available from: http://www.ncbi.nlm.nih.gov/pubmed/30255358.
9. Crofford LJ. Use of NSAIDs in treating patients with arthritis. Arthritis Res Ther [Internet]. 2013;15(Suppl 3):S2. Available from: http://www.ncbi.nlm.nih.gov/pubmed/24267197

Clinical Evaluation of Musculoskeletal Soft Tissue Complaints

2

Abstract

Soft tissue musculoskeletal complaints are extremely common in clinical practice and make up a significant portion of rheumatology referrals. While usually benign, these soft tissue syndromes can nevertheless cause significant pain and functional limitations and may even mimic more serious arthritic or systemic conditions. Careful evaluation helps distinguish benign, self-limiting conditions from those requiring urgent investigation. For patients, persistent soft tissue pain can diminish quality of life and productivity, so improving the evaluation and management of these complaints has tangible benefits. These cases require a thoughtful clinical assessment to distinguish mechanical, localised problems from inflammatory or systemic disorders. A careful history and physical examination remain the cornerstones of diagnosis, allowing the clinician to identify characteristic patterns and any "red flag" features that may signal a more serious pathology.

Case Scenario

A 38-year-old woman presents with 2 months of gradually worsening right shoulder pain. She has difficulty reaching overhead and finds it painful to put on a jacket, with aching that sometimes wakes her at night. She notes minimal morning stiffness and no noticeable swelling. On examination, there is tenderness around the shoulder tip and pain between 60° and 120° of arm abduction but nearly full passive range of motion.

© The Author(s), under exclusive license to Springer Nature Switzerland AG 2026
R. Amarnani, *Soft Tissue and Musculoskeletal Medicine in Rheumatology*,
https://doi.org/10.1007/978-3-032-29441-8_2

Analysis

These findings suggest rotator cuff-related shoulder pain, such as rotator cuff tendinopathy or subacromial pain syndrome, rather than glenohumeral joint arthritis, illustrating how history and exam guide the diagnosis. In this case, the absence of true joint swelling or prolonged stiffness, preservation of passive motion, and a painful mid-range arc of motion are hallmarks rotator cuff related shoulder pain. In contrast, if this were glenohumeral joint arthritis, one would expect restricted passive motion and possibly visible swelling or warmth. This example underscores how the clinical evaluation differentiates soft tissue issues from intraarticular pathology.

History and Symptom Evaluation

A detailed history often provides the majority of information needed to diagnose soft tissue rheumatologic conditions. The clinician should begin by characterising the patient's pain and symptoms thoroughly. Key aspects include the *onset* (sudden vs gradual), *duration* (acute vs chronic) and any precipitating *trauma or overuse.* An acute onset after a specific injury might suggest a sprain, strain or tear, whereas insidious onset without any clear trauma could indicate repetitive microtrauma or an underlying inflammatory process. Determine if the pain is *localised* to a specific structure or more *diffuse*. Patients can often point with one finger to a focal spot (e.g. the lateral elbow in epicondylitis) for soft tissue injuries, whereas articular (joint) pain may be more diffuse or deep-seated.

Evaluate the *quality* and *radiation* of the pain. Sharp, shooting pain or tingling that radiates might imply nerve involvement, whereas a dull, aching pain over a region could arise from muscle or tendon injury. Note any *diurnal pattern*. Pain that worsens with activity and improves with rest is typically mechanical. In contrast, pain from an inflammatory process tends to be worst after prolonged rest (e.g. prominent morning stiffness) and gradually improves as the day progresses. Ask about *morning stiffness*—stiffness lasting more than 30–60 minutes after waking strongly suggests an inflammatory condition (such as rheumatoid arthritis or polymyalgia rheumatica) rather than a purely mechanical complaint, where morning stiffness (if present at all) is usually brief (only a few minutes). Likewise, inflammatory pain may even *disturb sleep* in the second half of the night, whereas purely mechanical pain tends to hurt only with movement or at the end of a long day.

Inquire about any *swelling, redness or warmth* that the patient has noticed. True joint swelling suggests synovitis or effusion, whereas focal extra-articular swelling may indicate bursitis, tenosynovitis or other soft tissue inflammation. In contrast, many soft tissue pains (like tendinopathies) cause significant discomfort without obvious swelling. Identify any *mechanical factors*, for example, does the pain occur or worsen with certain motions, sports or occupational activities? A history of repetitive motions (such as heavy lifting, typing or running) can implicate specific overuse injuries. For instance, a carpenter with chronic elbow pain may develop lateral epicondylitis from hammering, or a new mother with radial wrist pain might have De Quervain's tenosynovitis from repeatedly lifting her infant. Also review the patient's *treatment response* so far—relief with rest or NSAIDs supports a mechanical or mild inflammatory issue, whereas only partial or no relief may occur in the setting of severe inflammation or other causes.

A comprehensive history should also screen for *systemic or constitutional symptoms*. Fever, unexplained weight loss, night sweats or profound fatigue accompanying musculoskeletal pain are red flags for infection, malignancy or a systemic rheumatic disease. Ask about *other joints or areas* of pain and any prolonged *morning stiffness* in joints aside from the primary complaint, which might suggest a generalised inflammatory disorder. For example, isolated shoulder girdle pain could be a localised soft tissue issue, but if the patient also describes prolonged morning stiffness and hip girdle aching, polymyalgia rheumatica should be considered. A history of *skin rashes, eye inflammation or bowel symptoms* is also relevant—such features might point towards a systemic condition like psoriatic arthritis or a spondyloarthritis if present alongside the soft tissue complaint.

Determining whether the pain is *articular (joint)* or *periarticular (soft tissue)* is a critical goal of the history. Clues include the exact location of pain and which movements provoke it. Pain exacerbated by *active motion* but not by passive motion often implicates a contractile structure (muscle or tendon), since the patient's own muscle activation is required to elicit pain. In contrast, true intraarticular pain typically occurs with both active and passive movements of the joint (e.g. both the patient moving their knee and the examiner moving it for them cause pain in knee arthritis). A complaint like "my knee hurts when going down stairs" might result from a patellar or quadriceps tendon issue if the pain is located at the front of the knee (load on the tendon increases with stairs), vs patellofemoral joint arthritis if there is a grinding sensation and pain deep in the joint. Clarifying these nuances in the history will guide a more focused physical examination.

It is also important to elicit any *neurologic symptoms* associated with the musculoskeletal complaint. Numbness, tingling or weakness may indicate nerve compression or radiculopathy rather than a primary soft tissue lesion. For example, lateral shoulder pain might suggest rotator cuff pathology, but if it is accompanied by numbness or shooting pain down the arm, one should consider cervical nerve root irritation as the true source. Similarly, low back or gluteal pain that radiates below the knee suggests nerve root involvement (e.g. lumbar radiculopathy) rather than a simple muscular strain.

Finally, the history should review any relevant *past medical history* and potential *risk factors*. Previous injuries or surgeries to the area can predispose to chronic soft tissue problems. Conditions like diabetes or obesity might influence tendon quality and healing capacity. Medication history is also useful; for instance, recent or repeated fluoroquinolone antibiotic exposure is a recognised risk factor for tendinopathy or tendon rupture, particularly in higher-risk patients. Some medications (such as statin therapy) can lead to diffuse muscle pain or weakness, and chronic corticosteroid use may contribute to tendon fragility. Also ask about any *family history* of rheumatic or autoimmune diseases, especially if you suspect a systemic condition. Finally, consider the *psychosocial context* of the pain. Determine how the musculoskeletal issue affects the patient's daily activities, work, sleep and mood. Chronic musculoskeletal pain can be exacerbated by stress, anxiety or misconceptions. Understanding the patient's concerns (e.g. the fear that a persistent pain signifies a serious illness) allows you to provide appropriate reassurance and education.

Throughout the history, the clinician should be constructing a working differential diagnosis. By the end of the interview, one should have hypotheses about whether the problem is likely mechanical or inflammatory, articular or soft tissue and which specific structures might be involved. This directs a more efficient and targeted physical examination.

Physical Examination

The physical examination of a patient with musculoskeletal complaints should be systematic and comparative. A *"look, feel, move"* approach is a time-honoured framework. Always examine the corresponding limb or region on the opposite side for comparison, to establish the patient's normal baseline. Additionally, examine the joint *above and below* the primary area of concern to ensure the pain is not referred from those sites (for instance, hip pathology can manifest as knee pain, or cervical spine issues can cause shoulder-region pain).

It is also crucial to observe general aspects of the patient's movement and posture. For example, note the patient's gait and how they sit or stand even before the focused exam begins. A quick general musculoskeletal screening examination such as the *GALS* (gait, arms, legs, spine) locomotor screen can be useful to catch any gross abnormalities [1]. This brief screening involves observing the patient's gait, asking them to perform simple movements of the arms and legs (including a full squat to assess lower limb function) and checking basic spinal motion.

Inspection

Begin the focused exam with careful inspection of the affected area. *Expose* the region adequately so that all relevant anatomy is visible (e.g. have the patient wear shorts for a knee exam or a gown that allows the shoulders and arms to be seen for a shoulder exam). Look for *swelling* or effusions. In a joint, an effusion may appear as fullness in the joint recesses (such as a bulge alongside the patella in a swollen knee), whereas in soft tissue, it may appear as a focal bulge (for instance, a fluid-filled lump over the olecranon in bursitis). Distinguish a diffuse joint swelling from a more localised swelling confined to a tendon sheath or bursal area. Note any *erythema* (redness) or other skin changes. Redness and warmth suggest active inflammation or infection (e.g. a cellulitic area over a tendon sheath or an acutely inflamed bursitis). Also check for *bruising* (ecchymosis); bruising around a joint or muscle can indicate a recent acute injury such as a tear or significant strain.

Next, assess the *contour and symmetry* of the musculature around the affected region. *Muscle wasting* or atrophy may develop with chronic joint dysfunction or after a tendon rupture—for example, a long-standing rotator cuff tear can lead to visible thinning of the shoulder muscles (supraspinatus and infraspinatus areas). Compare muscle bulk side to side; significant asymmetry can indicate disuse atrophy or even a motor nerve lesion affecting that muscle group. Conversely, *swelling or hypertrophy* of soft tissues can be seen in certain chronic conditions (for instance, the Achilles tendon may appear thickened in chronic tendinosis). Look at the *alignment* of the joint and limb. Is there any deformity or abnormal posture? For example, a patient with a large knee effusion often holds the knee in slight flexion for comfort, and a person with a long-standing tendon injury might exhibit an abnormal posture to offload the painful structure. A collapsed foot arch might indicate posterior tibial tendon dysfunction, while an excessive kyphosis or scoliosis in the spine might become apparent on inspection. Check if the shoulders are level or if one is drooping—unilateral trapezius muscle wasting or spinal curvature can cause asymmetry.

During inspection, also pay attention to how the patient *moves* the affected area spontaneously. Are they guarding or avoiding certain motions? For instance, with a painful shoulder, the patient may keep the arm tucked against the body and have reduced arm swing when walking. In lower limb injuries, observe the gait: there may be an obvious limp, an unwillingness to bear weight fully on one side or a shortened stance phase on the affected limb (antalgic gait). These subtle cues—noted even before formal testing—can provide clues about the severity and nature of the problem.

Palpation

After inspection, proceed to *palpation*, which helps identify tender structures and assess for warmth or swelling in the area. Palpate *systematically* over the bones, joints and soft tissues of the region. Ask the patient to point to the area of maximum pain, and then gently palpate that spot and the surrounding structures to localise the *tenderness*. Localised tenderness at a specific tendon insertion or along a muscle belly can confirm a suspected tendinopathy or muscle strain. For example, marked tenderness at the lateral epicondyle strongly supports the diagnosis of lateral epicondylitis (tennis elbow) if that was suspected from the history. Palpation can also reveal *thickening or crepitus* in tendon sheaths; for instance, a creaking sensation felt over the wrist extensors might be noted in severe De Quervain's tenosynovitis.

Use the back of your hand to compare *temperature* between the affected area and the opposite side. Even a slight increase in warmth over a joint or tendon can signify active inflammation. While palpating around joints, try to detect any *effusion*. In the knee, for example, one can attempt a bulge sign or patellar tap to confirm the presence of excess fluid in the joint. In an elbow or shoulder, an effusion is harder to discern by touch, but look for subtle fullness in the normal recesses. Remember that many soft tissue conditions do not cause true joint effusions—the absence of detectable intraarticular fluid can support a periarticular diagnosis rather than an internal joint pathology.

Evaluate the *muscle tone* and check for areas of muscle spasm. In cases like low back strain or cervical strain, palpation often reveals taut muscle bands or *trigger points* in the paraspinal or shoulder girdle muscles; pressing on these can reproduce the patient's pain (a classic feature of myofascial pain syndrome). Note any *fibrous nodules* or gaps in structures: a palpable defect in a tendon (e.g. a gap in the Achilles tendon about 4–6 cm above the heel) is highly suggestive of a complete tendon rupture. Likewise, tenderness directly at tendon or ligament attachments on bone (the *entheses*) can indicate an enthesitis (inflammatory tendon insertion disease), as is seen in the spondyloarthritis (for instance, a very tender Achilles tendon insertion in a patient with suspected reactive arthritis).

If appropriate, palpate related or adjacent structures to evaluate for referred pain. For example, in a patient with shoulder pain, palpating the neck (cervical spine and musculature) can reveal that the pain might actually stem from cervical radiculopathy rather than the shoulder itself. In a patient complaining of lateral hip pain, palpating the lumbar spine and sacroiliac joints can help determine if the discomfort is referred from the lower back. Similarly, palpating regional lymph node basins (such as the inguinal nodes in a patient with thigh or knee swelling) could uncover lymphadenopathy suggestive of infection or tumour that might otherwise be overlooked.

Range of Motion

Assess the patient's *range of motion (ROM)* next. Test *active ROM* first by having the patient move the joint or limb through its full range. Observe for any limitation in movement or reproduction of pain. If active motion is limited or painful, gently test the joint's *passive ROM* by moving it for the patient (while they relax) to see if the range can be achieved without their muscular effort. Compare the findings: if a joint's movement is restricted both actively and passively, this suggests an intrinsic joint problem (such as significant arthritis, a contracture or a large effusion limiting the joint's mobility). In contrast, if passive motion is normal (or significantly greater than active motion) and is less painful than active movement, a soft tissue issue involving the muscles or tendons is more likely—because those tissues are not being strained during passive movement. For example, a patient with a large rotator cuff tear may be unable to actively lift the arm overhead, but the examiner can passively lift it to near-normal range (a classic "drop arm" scenario). Conversely, in adhesive capsulitis of the shoulder (a frozen shoulder), both active and passive motion are markedly restricted in a capsular pattern.

Document the degree of motion achieved, either quantitatively (in degrees, if goniometry is available) or qualitatively (e.g. "full", "slightly limited", "half normal range"). Note whether any motion causes *crepitus* or instability. A palpable or audible *crepitus* (grinding or crackling) during movement suggests roughened articular surfaces as seen in osteoarthritis or may come from tendons snapping over bony prominences in conditions like tendinitis. *Instability* on movement—an excessive looseness of a joint—indicates possible ligamentous laxity or tear. For instance, an anterior cruciate ligament tear in the knee can lead to anterior instability (the tibia slides forward too much relative to the femur). If any instability is observed or suspected, specific stability tests (described below) should be performed to further evaluate the integrity of the ligaments.

It is also helpful to assess *functional movements* as part of the ROM evaluation. Ask the patient to perform motions that mimic daily activities or aggravating movements. For a shoulder problem, can the patient reach up to comb their hair or reach behind their back to fasten clothing? For a lower extremity issue, can they rise from a chair without using their arms, squat down or go up on their toes? Observing these functional tasks can reveal deficits that matter to the patient's quality of life and may elicit pain at specific points in the motion. For example, a patient with shoulder impingement might have pain reaching overhead or a painful arc between 60° and 120° of abduction.

Additionally, assess for *generalised joint hypermobility* by looking for signs such as elbow hyperextension, knee hyperextension, the ability to touch the thumbs to the forearm and excessive finger extension (elements of the Beighton score). A significant degree of hypermobility (present in 2–57% of adults) [2] may predispose individuals to soft tissue injuries. If your patient is notably hypermobile (e.g. can easily place their palms flat on the floor or hyperextend their knees by 10°), this laxity could be contributing to recurrent sprains or joint pains, and it is an important factor to consider in management.

Special Tests

After completing the general examination, perform any region-specific *special tests* that can help confirm your diagnostic suspicions. Special tests are targeted manoeuvres designed to stress particular structures or reproduce specific symptoms. For example, if lateral epicondylitis (tennis elbow) is suspected, *Cozen's test* (resisted wrist extension with the elbow extended) will provoke pain at the lateral epicondyle when positive [3]. For shoulder impingement, tests like the *Neer impingement sign* (passive forward elevation of the arm causing subacromial pain) or the *Hawkins-Kennedy test* (forward elevation of the arm to 90° with forced internal rotation) can reproduce the patient's shoulder pain [4]. In suspected carpal tunnel syndrome (median nerve compression at the wrist), manoeuvres such as *Tinel's sign* (tapping over the median nerve at the wrist to elicit tingling in the hand) or *Phalen's test* (maximally flexing the wrists together for 60 seconds to provoke symptoms) are classically used [5]. Likewise, if it is unclear whether shoulder pain might actually be referred from a cervical nerve root, a *Spurling's test* (extension and rotation of the neck with downward pressure on the head) can reproduce radicular arm pain, indicating a cervical spine origin rather than a shoulder joint problem [6].

Each area of the body has its own repertoire of special manoeuvres; the clinician should choose those that correspond to the leading hypotheses from the history and initial exam. A positive result on a special test can bolster confidence in a diagnosis, whereas a negative result may prompt reconsideration of other causes. Keep in mind that no single special test is perfectly sensitive or specific—their diagnostic utility varies—so these findings must be interpreted within the broader clinical context. Often, a *combination of tests* yields the best accuracy. For instance, in the shoulder, a combination of positive Neer, Hawkins and painful arc tests strongly points towards subacromial impingement syndrome. In addition to these provocative manoeuvres, assess related factors such as muscle strength and joint stability. If you suspect a tendon tear, evaluate the strength of the corresponding muscle group (e.g. significant weakness in external rotation of the shoulder suggests a possible rotator cuff tear involving the infraspinatus). Perform *ligament stability tests* for joints where a sprain or ligament tear is in the differential, for example, applying varus and valgus stress to a painful knee to test the collateral ligaments or doing an anterior drawer test on an injured ankle to check for lateral ligament laxity. Pain or excessive laxity on these stress tests confirms ligamentous injury. All special test results should be integrated with the rest of the examination to ensure a correct interpretation.

Finally, ensure a basic *neurologic examination* is conducted when appropriate. Check the key muscle groups for strength, assess pertinent reflexes and test sensory function in the affected limb. Even if the primary complaint appears to be musculoskeletal, subtle neurologic deficits can change your diagnostic thinking or urgency of referral. For example, slight weakness in ankle dorsiflexion or a loss of the ankle reflex in a patient with leg pain might indicate an L5/S1 radiculopathy, changing a presumed localised tendon problem into a spine issue requiring further workup. Detecting such signs early is crucial, as they may necessitate prompt imaging or specialist intervention (e.g. for potential nerve compression).

Red Flag Signs

While most soft tissue musculoskeletal complaints are benign and self-limited, it is imperative to recognise certain *red flags* that indicate a potentially serious condition requiring urgent evaluation or referral. Be alert for the following:

- *Constitutional symptoms:* Fever, chills, night sweats or unexplained weight loss accompanying musculoskeletal pain. These systemic signs raise concern for underlying infection (e.g. septic arthritis or osteomyelitis) or malignancy as a cause of the pain.
- *Persistent night pain or pain at rest:* Pain that is unrelenting and present even during rest, especially if it wakes the patient from sleep, is atypical for benign mechanical issues. Such a pattern suggests possible tumour involvement (a bone malignancy or metastasis) or an infection (such as osteomyelitis) and warrants prompt investigation.
- *Hot, red, swollen joint or soft tissue:* An intensely inflamed, warm and erythematous joint suggests septic arthritis until proven otherwise. Similarly, a red, swollen bursa or soft tissue (like a very tender, red olecranon) raises concern for septic bursitis or cellulitis. This presentation strongly suggests an urgent process

(infection or acute crystal arthritis like gout) that requires immediate diagnostic aspiration and treatment.

- *Significant weakness or neurological deficits:* Objective motor or sensory deficits (e.g. foot drop or numbness in a dermatomal distribution) in the context of musculoskeletal pain indicate possible nerve compression or central neurologic involvement. For example, new ankle dorsiflexion weakness in a patient with leg pain may indicate L5 radiculopathy or another significant neuropathic process. Bilateral neurological symptoms, saddle anaesthesia or bladder/bowel dysfunction should raise concern for cauda equina syndrome [7]. Neurologic red flags often warrant emergent imaging and specialist referral.
- *History of malignancy or immune suppression:* A patient with a known prior cancer who develops new bone or soft tissue pain should be evaluated for possible skeletal metastases. Likewise, an immunosuppressed patient (on biologics, chemotherapy or high-dose steroids) presenting with localised musculoskeletal pain is at higher risk for unusual infections (such as fungal or atypical bacterial infections) in bones or joints.
- *Trauma with deformity or loss of function:* Significant trauma followed by inability to bear weight or a visible deformity of a limb suggests a fracture or dislocation. Even if a patient assumes it is "just a sprain," a high-energy injury mechanism with such findings should be treated as a possible fracture until proven otherwise by imaging.
- *Multiple sites of pain with disproportionate tenderness:* Widespread pain accompanied by extreme tenderness at many sites (in the absence of objective swelling or inflammation) is more suggestive of fibromyalgia or a centralised pain syndrome than of an acute anatomic lesion. While not a red flag for dangerous disease, recognising this pattern prevents exhaustive (and unnecessary) searches for a focal inflammatory or malignant cause and guides appropriate management of the pain syndrome.

Whenever red flag features are present, further diagnostic workup (imaging, laboratory tests) should be promptly arranged, and referral to an appropriate specialist should be considered. Conversely, in the absence of red flags, the evaluation can usually proceed in a more routine manner and one can be more conservative about ordering extensive tests initially.

Distinguishing Mechanical Versus Inflammatory Pain

Broadly, musculoskeletal pain complaints can be categorised as predominantly *mechanical* or *inflammatory* in nature. It is far more common to encounter mechanical soft tissue pain than true inflammatory pathology in everyday practice, but identifying the latter is critical to ensure appropriate therapy and to avoid missing serious disease.

A key outcome of the clinical evaluation is deciding whether a patient's pain is due to a mechanical cause or an inflammatory process. The typical *clinical patterns* of mechanical and inflammatory pain differ:

- *Mechanical pain:* This type of musculoskeletal pain is related to activity or biomechanical stress on tissues. It tends to *worsen with exercise or towards the end of the day* and *improves with rest*. Morning stiffness, if present, is brief (typically *<30 minutes*). Mechanical pain often arises from degenerative changes, overuse or minor injuries affecting soft tissues (e.g. osteoarthritis, tendinopathy, ligament sprain). Swelling is usually mild or localised, and *systemic symptoms* are absent. Laboratory tests (e.g. inflammatory markers) are typically normal. A classic example is knee osteoarthritis causing pain after prolonged walking or standing but little to no stiffness in the morning. On examination, mechanical lesions may have localised tenderness and pain with movement but no significant warmth or redness.
- *Inflammatory pain* [8]*:* Inflammatory pain from immune-mediated arthritis often improves with activity and worsens after rest. Crystal arthritis, such as acute gout, is also inflammatory but typically presents as abrupt severe pain, often with marked rest pain and exquisite tenderness. It characteristically *improves with activity* and *worsens after periods of rest.* Patients often report prominent *morning stiffness* that lasts *>30–60 minutes* (sometimes several hours) after waking. Inflammatory pain may also *wake the patient at night,* especially in the early morning hours. There are often objective signs of inflammation: *swelling, warmth and sometimes erythema* of the affected joints or tissues. *Systemic features* like fatigue, low-grade fever or other organ involvement can be present in systemic rheumatic diseases [9]. Laboratory tests frequently show elevated acute phase reactants (e.g. ESR, CRP) or other markers of inflammation. A prime example is rheumatoid arthritis, where patients have prolonged morning stiffness, symmetric joint swelling and improved symptoms with movement as the day goes on. Another example is an acute gout flare in which a patient has a red, hot, swollen big toe that is extremely painful at rest or at night. On examination, an inflamed joint or tendon sheath will be very tender even to gentle passive movement, and there may be diffuse tenderness beyond just one focal point.

Some soft tissue rheumatologic conditions can have both mechanical and inflammatory components. For instance, chronic degenerative tendinopathy can have episodes of reactive inflammation, and conversely a patient with an inflammatory arthritis can suffer a mechanical tendon tear. Furthermore, patients may have concurrent mechanical and inflammatory issues. For example, an individual with rheumatoid arthritis (inflammatory) might also develop a rotator cuff tear or tendinopathy (mechanical); each condition will contribute its own pain pattern and must be evaluated in context. Nonetheless, categorising the predominant pain pattern as mechanical vs inflammatory is very helpful. If clear inflammatory features are present, the threshold for further investigation (imaging, lab tests) and rheumatology referral is lower. If the pattern is entirely mechanical, one might manage conservatively and observe response to treatment before pursuing extensive workups.

Key Learning Points

- A thorough *history and physical exam* are usually sufficient to diagnose the majority of musculoskeletal soft tissue complaints. Careful attention to symptom patterns (timing, triggers, alleviating factors) and exam findings (location of tenderness, effect of movement, etc.) is crucial for accurate diagnosis.
- *Distinguish articular vs soft tissue pain:* Articular (joint) pain typically causes pain with any movement and often presents with joint swelling or loss of passive motion, whereas soft tissue pain is often localised to a particular tendon, bursa or muscle and causes pain mainly during specific movements or positions that stress the affected structure.
- *Mechanical vs inflammatory patterns:* Mechanical soft tissue pain (e.g. degenerative or overuse conditions) tends to worsen with activity and improve with rest, with minimal morning stiffness. Inflammatory pain (as seen in systemic rheumatic diseases or acute crystal arthritis) tends to improve with activity and worsen after rest, often with significant morning stiffness and obvious signs of inflammation.
- Always screen for *red flag* signs (fever, weight loss, severe night/rest pain, neurologic deficits, history of cancer, etc.). Their presence should prompt urgent evaluation for infection, malignancy, fracture or other serious pathology rather than a simple soft tissue injury.
- The musculoskeletal examination should be *systematic*: inspect for visible abnormalities; palpate for tenderness, swelling or warmth; assess range of motion (active and passive); and perform special tests targeted to the suspected diagnosis. Always compare findings with the contralateral side and consider the patient's normal baseline.
- *Most soft tissue diagnoses are clinical.* Imaging and laboratory tests play only a supportive role when indicated. In the absence of red flags, a well-conducted history and exam often suffice for diagnosis and should guide the use of any further investigations.

References

1. Plant MJ, Linton S, Dodd E, Jones PW, Dawes PT. The GALS locomotor screen and disability. Ann Rheum Dis [Internet]. 1993;52(12):886–90. Available from: http://www.ncbi.nlm.nih.gov/pubmed/8311541
2. Blajwajs L, Williams J, Timmons W, Sproule J. Hypermobility prevalence, measurements, and outcomes in childhood, adolescence, and emerging adulthood: a systematic review. Rheumatol Int [Internet]. 2023;43(8):1423–44. Available from: http://www.ncbi.nlm.nih.gov/pubmed/37149553
3. Soares MM, Souza PC, Ribeiro AP. Differences in clinical tests for assessing lateral epicondylitis elbow in adults concerning their physical activity level: test reliability, accuracy of ultrasound imaging, and relationship with energy expenditure. Int J Environ Res Public Health [Internet]. 2023;20(3) Available from: http://www.ncbi.nlm.nih.gov/pubmed/36767167

4. Tennent TD, Beach WR, Meyers JF. A review of the special tests associated with shoulder examination. Part I: the rotator cuff tests. Am J Sports Med [Internet]. 2003;31(1):154–60. Available from: http://www.ncbi.nlm.nih.gov/pubmed/12531773
5. Roghani AS, Farooq J, Ullah W, Roghani FS, Ahmad B, Jan AA, et al. Diagnostic accuracy of clinical examination for carpal tunnel syndrome: validation using nerve conduction studies. Cureus [Internet]. 2025;17(7):e87563. Available from: http://www.ncbi.nlm.nih.gov/pubmed/40786347
6. Jones SJ, Miller J-MM. Spurling test [Internet]. In: StatPearls; 2026. Available from: http://www.ncbi.nlm.nih.gov/pubmed/29228289.
7. Miller J, West J, Khawar H, Middleton R. Cauda equina syndrome. Br J Hosp Med (Lond) [Internet]. 2023;84(11):1–7. Available from: http://www.ncbi.nlm.nih.gov/pubmed/38186331
8. Khot S, Tackley G, Choy E. How to distinguish non-inflammatory from inflammatory pain in RA? Curr Rheumatol Rep [Internet]. 2024;26(12):403–13. Available from: http://www.ncbi.nlm.nih.gov/pubmed/39120749
9. Cheikh M, Bahabri N. Fever and rheumatology [Internet]. In: Skills in rheumatology; 2021. Available from: https://www.ncbi.nlm.nih.gov/books/NBK585733/.

Diagnostic Tools: Imaging and Investigations

3

Abstract

Diagnostic evaluation in soft tissue and musculoskeletal rheumatology relies on a combination of targeted imaging and laboratory investigations to clarify the clinical picture. This chapter reviews the role of imaging modalities—including ultrasound, MRI, CT and X-ray—in diagnosing soft tissue rheumatic conditions, emphasising when to use each test based on clinical presentation. Strengths and limitations of each modality are discussed, with specific examples such as tendon tears, bursitis, calcific tendinitis and enthesopathies illustrating key imaging findings (normal vs pathological). The integration of laboratory tests (e.g. ESR, CRP, autoimmune serologies, urate) is also explored, highlighting when blood tests or synovial fluid analysis can confirm or exclude systemic inflammatory conditions underlying a soft tissue complaint. A practical diagnostic algorithm is provided to guide clinicians in selecting appropriate investigations, recognising "red flag" signs that warrant urgent imaging and interpreting results in context.

Case Vignette

Case

A 46-year-old construction worker presents with chronic lateral elbow pain and intermittent swelling. Conservative treatments for presumed "tennis elbow" (lateral epicondylitis) have provided little relief. On exam, there is localised tenderness over the common extensor tendon origin but also mild warmth and a small effusion at the lateral epicondyle. There is no obvious synovitis or loss of elbow range of motion. Given the persistent symptoms and atypical exam findings, the clinician faces a diagnostic dilemma: *Is this simply a refractory tendinopathy, or could an underlying systemic or structural pathology be present?* The challenge is determining which diagnostic tools, imaging and/or laboratory tests, could help confirm the diagnosis. Should an ultrasound be done to evaluate the extensor tendon and bursa

© The Author(s), under exclusive license to Springer Nature Switzerland AG 2026

R. Amarnani, *Soft Tissue and Musculoskeletal Medicine in Rheumatology*,
https://doi.org/10.1007/978-3-032-29441-8_3

or perhaps an X-ray to look for calcifications or bony changes? Would inflammatory markers, rheumatoid factor and anti-CCP be useful if the history or examination suggested an inflammatory arthritis? This case highlights the uncertainty in choosing and interpreting *imaging and investigations* for soft tissue rheumatic complaints. In the following sections, we will explore how a clinician can systematically approach such diagnostic challenges using the available tools.

Role of Imaging in Soft Tissue Rheumatology

Imaging is an invaluable extension of the clinical examination for soft tissue rheumatic disorders. Many soft tissue conditions—tendinopathies, bursitis, enthesopathies, etc.—involve structures that are not directly visible or palpable, and imaging can confirm clinical suspicions, assess severity and sometimes reveal unexpected pathology. For example, in the case above, appropriate imaging might differentiate a simple lateral epicondylar tendinopathy from an occult olecranon bursitis or intraarticular pathology. Generally, *imaging should be guided by clinical findings:* it is most useful when the diagnosis is uncertain, when confirming the extent of an injury or when looking for features that would change management (such as a tendon tear requiring surgical repair). Unnecessary imaging should be avoided in straightforward cases to prevent incidental findings and excess cost.

In soft tissue rheumatology, the main imaging modalities include *ultrasound, magnetic resonance imaging (MRI), computed tomography (CT) and plain radiography (X-rays)* [1]. Each modality has a distinct role. Plain X-rays are often used as a *first-line screening* to detect fractures, degenerative joint changes or calcific deposits, given their wide availability and low cost [2]. Ultrasound has become a frontline tool because it allows dynamic, real-time examination of tendons, bursae and entheses and can be done at the point of care. MRI provides comprehensive detail of soft tissues and bone marrow, useful for complex or deep structures not easily seen on ultrasound. CT is less commonly needed in soft tissue rheumatology but can delineate calcifications or bone involvement when MRI is contraindicated. Importantly, each modality's *strengths and limitations* must be considered. In the sections below, we give an overview of each imaging tool and provide guidance on selecting the right test for various clinical scenarios.

Imaging Modalities in Soft Tissue Rheumatology

Ultrasound [3]

Ultrasound (US) is a cornerstone of soft tissue imaging in rheumatology due to its high resolution for superficial structures, lack of radiation and ability to perform *dynamic and comparative examinations*. Modern high-frequency musculoskeletal ultrasound can visualise tendons, ligaments, bursae and even small joints with great detail. It excels at detecting *tendon abnormalities* (tendinosis, tears), effusions and bursitis and *enthesitis* (inflammation at tendon insertions). Additionally, Doppler ultrasound can assess blood flow as an indicator of active inflammation (e.g. synovial or entheseal hyperaemia) [4]. A major advantage is that ultrasound can be used *in real time* during the physical exam, for example, the patient can point to the area of pain, and the clinician can directly visualise the underlying structure while moving the limb.

Strengths Ultrasound is *highly sensitive* for many soft tissue lesions and has been shown to have diagnostic accuracy comparable to MRI for certain conditions, notably rotator cuff tears [5]. For instance, meta-analyses have found that ultrasound and MRI both have >90% sensitivity and specificity for full-thickness rotator cuff tears [5], and ultrasound is similarly effective in detecting high-grade tendon injuries (with somewhat lower sensitivity for small partial tears). Given its *low cost and convenience*, experts often recommend ultrasound as a first-line imaging test for rotator cuff pathology, especially when performed by experienced providers [6]. Ultrasound also allows *dynamic assessment,* for example, one can observe a snapping tendon or impingement by moving the joint during the scan and can evaluate the contralateral side for comparison. Another practical benefit is that ultrasound can guide interventions: the clinician can precisely guide needle aspirations or corticosteroid injections into bursae, tendon sheaths or around calcific deposits under direct visualisation.

Limitations The main limitation of ultrasound is that it is *operator-dependent* [7]—the accuracy heavily relies on the skill and experience of the person performing the scan. Structures that are deep or obscured by bone are not well seen on ultrasound. For example, ultrasound cannot visualise through bone and provides only a limited assessment of deeper intra-articular structures; it cannot assess bone marrow oedema [8]. In the spine or pelvis (e.g. sacroiliac joints), ultrasound has virtually no role. Additionally, patients with greater soft tissue depth or areas with extensive soft tissue may be challenging due to limited penetration of high-frequency probes. Despite these limitations, in the hands of a skilled clinician, ultrasound provides an excellent combination of *diagnostic accuracy, safety and immediacy* for many soft tissue rheumatic conditions.

Magnetic Resonance Imaging (MRI)

MRI is often considered the most comprehensive modality for musculoskeletal soft tissue assessment. It uses strong magnetic fields and radiofrequency pulses to generate high-resolution images with excellent soft tissue contrast. MRI can visualise not only tendons and muscles but also articular cartilage, ligaments, bone marrow and even small subtle features like oedema or synovial hypertrophy. In soft tissue rheumatology, MRI is particularly valuable for *complex or deep regions* and when a comprehensive assessment is needed.

Strengths MRI provides a *multiplanar view* of anatomy with unparalleled contrast resolution for soft tissues. It can detect changes that other modalities miss—for example, bone marrow oedema (an early sign of stress injury or enthesitis in spondyloarthritis) is clearly seen on MRI but not on X-ray [9]. MRI is very useful for confirming and staging *muscle or tendon tears* (e.g. differentiating partial vs full-thickness rotator cuff tears or detecting retraction of a torn tendon). It is also sensitive for *inflammation*; active inflammatory changes in both soft tissue and bone (such as tenosynovitis, osteitis or bursitis) show characteristic signal changes on MRI (like T2-weighted fluid signal and postcontrast enhancement) [10]. In settings where ultrasound might be limited—for instance, evaluating a deep structure like the hip tendons or intraarticular soft tissue—MRI is often the next step. Importantly, MRI does not use ionising radiation, making it safer for repeated use and for younger patients [11].

Limitations [11] The downsides of MRI include *cost, availability and patient contraindications*. MRI is expensive and not as readily available as X-ray or ultrasound in many centres, often requiring scheduling and sometimes travel to specialised facilities. Scan times are longer (typically 20–40 minutes per region), and patients must remain very still; this can be an issue for those in pain or with claustrophobia. Certain patients cannot undergo MRI, such as those with incompatible implanted devices (pacemakers, some cochlear implants, etc.) or severe claustrophobia (though open MRIs or sedation can mitigate this in some cases). Compared to ultrasound, MRI is *less accessible at the bedside*—it is usually a second-line test after simpler modalities. Another limitation is that MRI may detect *incidental findings* that are not clinically significant, potentially complicating the picture (e.g. asymptomatic degenerative changes in tendons or spine are common on MRI). Additionally, MRI's resolution for very fine superficial details can actually be slightly lower than a focused ultrasound. For example, small calcifications in a tendon are better detected on X-ray or ultrasound; on MRI, they appear as nonspecific low-signal foci that could be missed [12]. Finally, MRI is generally not as good as CT for visualising cortical bone detail or calcific deposits (where CT or X-ray excel). In summary, MRI is *best reserved for cases requiring a comprehensive internal view* of the musculoskeletal area, particularly if initial tests are inconclusive or if serious pathology is suspected.

Computed Tomography (CT)

CT uses X-rays and computer processing to create cross-sectional images. In soft tissue rheumatology, CT is not routinely the first choice for most soft tissue conditions, but it has specific niche uses. CT excels at visualising *bony structures* in high detail and can detect calcifications well. It is often utilised when MRI is contraindicated or when precise bony anatomy is needed.

Strengths The primary advantage of CT is its superior visualisation of *bone and calcific densities* [13]. Tiny fractures (e.g. osteochondral fragments, stress fractures) or complex anatomical regions of bone can be delineated by CT when plain radiographs are insufficient. For instance, if there is a suspicion of a bone spur contributing to tendon impingement, CT can show the exact size and shape of the spur. CT can also help in characterising calcific tendinitis deposits if needed, as it will show them as high-density foci and can even produce three-dimensional reconstructions of their location [13]. CT scans are relatively quick (minutes) and widely available. In emergency situations (e.g. suspected fracture or bone involvement with inability to get MRI rapidly), CT can provide critical information. CT is also useful for guiding certain interventional procedures, though in rheumatology, this is less common (ultrasound or fluoroscopy is more often used for injections and biopsies, respectively).

Limitations [14] The limitations of CT are significant in the context of soft tissue evaluation. First, CT *involves radiation exposure*, which is a concern especially for younger patients or repeated imaging. Soft tissue contrast on CT is poorer than MRI—muscles, tendons and ligaments can be seen, but subtle differentiation (like oedema or inflammation) is usually not possible without intravenous contrast, and even then, MRI is superior. As a result, CT is *not ideal for detecting early inflammatory or soft tissue changes* unless they involve calcification or bone. MRI would, for example, identify a subtle tendon tear or synovitis that CT could easily miss if no calcification or gross structural change is present. Additionally, artifacts from metal (like joint replacements or surgical screws) can affect CT images (though MRI is often more severely affected by metal artifacts). In summary, CT's role in soft tissue rheumatology is limited; it is *generally reserved for scenarios where bone detail is crucial or MRI cannot be performed.* For most soft tissue diagnoses, ultrasound or MRI will be more informative.

Plain Radiography (X-Rays)

Conventional radiographs (X-rays) remain an essential diagnostic tool in musculoskeletal medicine. While X-rays primarily show bones, they also can reveal certain soft tissue clues and are often done as an initial imaging study. In rheumatology clinics, it is common to obtain X-rays to *exclude fractures, arthritis or gross abnormalities* when evaluating a regional pain complaint.

Strengths [15] X-rays are *quick, inexpensive and widely available*. They provide a high-level overview of the skeletal anatomy, which is important since soft tissue pain may sometimes be referred from a bone or joint problem. For example, a patient presenting with shoulder pain might get a shoulder X-ray first—this can show calcific deposits in tendons, acromial spurs (which could impinge on rotator cuff tendons) or glenohumeral joint space narrowing (suggesting osteoarthritis) that could be contributing to symptoms. In many cases, an X-ray helps *narrow the* *differential diagnosis* by distinguishing purely soft tissue causes from bony pathology. Certain soft tissue conditions have characteristic X-ray findings: *calcific tendinitis* is a prime example—calcium hydroxyapatite deposits within tendons (often in the rotator cuff) appear as homogeneous, amorphous dense opacities on X-ray. Enthesophytes (bony spurs at tendon insertions) are also visible on X-rays, reflecting chronic enthesopathy. X-rays can incidentally show soft tissue swelling or masses if large enough and on occasion gas in tissues (which would signal possible infection like necrotising fasciitis) or foreign bodies.

Limitations [16] The chief limitation is that X-rays have *limited sensitivity for soft tissue lesions* that do not involve calcification or bone changes. A normal X-ray does *not* rule out tendon tears, mild bursitis or early inflammatory changes. Soft tissues themselves are mostly not visualised; for instance, a rotator cuff tear will not be seen on X-ray unless it is chronic enough to cause secondary changes like proximal humeral migration or degeneration of the greater tuberosity. Similarly, a normal knee X-ray does not exclude a meniscal or ligamentous injury. Another limitation is radiation exposure, although the dose from an extremity or joint X-ray is quite low (much lower than CT). Nonetheless, avoiding unnecessary radiation is always a consideration, especially in younger patients. *Technique and views* matter as well—a single view can miss findings; multiple views or special positions are often needed (e.g. an outlet view of the shoulder to detect subacromial spurs). In summary, X-rays are *most useful as an initial survey* to catch any obvious bony abnormalities or calcifications and to guide further imaging. They are often normal in soft tissue rheumatic conditions, so further imaging is usually pursued if clinical suspicion remains high despite unremarkable X-rays.

Choosing the Right Imaging Test Based on Clinical Presentation

Given the array of imaging modalities, an important clinical skill is selecting the *appropriate test for each scenario*. The choice depends on factors such as the suspected diagnosis, the anatomical location, availability of imaging modalities and urgency. Below are general guidelines and examples to help choose wisely:

- *Start with plain X-ray if bone or calcification involvement is suspected:* If the patient's history or exam suggests a possible fracture, osteoarthritis or calcific deposit, an X-ray is often the first step. For example, in a patient with chronic shoulder pain, a plain radiograph can reveal calcific tendinitis or arthritis. In acute traumatic injuries (falls, sports injuries), X-ray is essential to rule out fractures. If an X-ray shows significant findings (like a large calcific deposit or joint degeneration), it may confirm the diagnosis without need for more expensive tests.
- *Use ultrasound for superficial soft tissue structures and dynamic assessment:* Ultrasound is usually the preferred initial advanced imaging for *tendon and*

bursa evaluations, especially in accessible areas like the shoulder, elbow, wrist, knee, ankle and foot. In a case of suspected *rotator cuff tear* without trauma, one might choose an ultrasound first to confirm the tear. Ultrasound is also useful for superficial tendon disorders such as lateral epicondylopathy and De Quervain's tenosynovitis, and for selected peripheral nerve entrapments such as carpal tunnel syndrome. If a patient has a localised swelling that could be a ganglion or bursitis, ultrasound can immediately determine if it is fluid-filled and even guide an aspiration. *Example:* Our case patient with lateral elbow pain—an ultrasound could visualise the common extensor tendon (to check for tendinosis or tears) and the olecranon area (to see if a bursitis or synovitis is present). This information might spare the patient an unnecessary MRI. Ultrasound is highly operator-dependent, so ensure the examiner is experienced in musculoskeletal scanning for reliable results.

- *Reserve MRI for deep structures, complex cases or surgical planning:* If initial imaging is inconclusive or the problem involves deep or multistructural pathology, MRI is often indicated. For instance, *hip girdle pain* in an obese patient might be evaluated with MRI if ultrasound is unable to adequately penetrate to the hip tendons or bursae. MRI is also indicated when *serious pathology is suspected*: for example, if one suspects osteomyelitis, occult fracture or a tumour masquerading as a soft tissue complaint, MRI (often with contrast) provides the necessary detail. Additionally, when surgical intervention is being considered (such as a rotator cuff repair), MRI can map out the full extent of injury (retraction of tendon, muscle atrophy, etc.) to aid surgical planning. For example, a middle-aged runner with chronic heel pain not responding to treatment might get an MRI if we suspect a partial *Achilles tendon tear* or plantar fascia tear that was not confirmed on ultrasound or to detect bone marrow oedema indicative of a stress fracture or spondyloarthropathy-related enthesitis.
- *CT as a problem-solver:* CT is usually not first-line for soft tissue rheumatologic issues, but think of it in specific scenarios: (1) when an MRI is needed but cannot be done (e.g. patient with pacemaker who presents with suspected pelvic stress fracture or sacroiliitis—a CT could at least show sclerosis or erosion, though it will not show inflammation as MRI would) and (2) when evaluating known calcific or osseous abnormalities in more detail. For *example,* in calcific tendinitis of the shoulder, if the calcium deposit is unusually located or an interventional radiologist needs to plan an ultrasound-guided needling, a prior CT could delineate the deposit's exact three-dimensional position (this is rarely necessary, however, as ultrasound itself usually suffices for guidance). In summary, CT is chosen only in select cases, often after consideration of the above modalities.
- *Combine imaging with clinical correlation:* Always interpret imaging results in light of the patient's clinical picture. A classic teaching is that *imaging should answer a specific question* posed by the clinical evaluation. For example, "Does this patient with shoulder pain have a rotator cuff tear or just tendinopathy?" If the ultrasound or MRI says "partial tear," correlate that with the patient's strength and exam; a small partial tear on MRI might not be the actual pain generator if the exam suggests otherwise or it might be an incidental age-related finding.

Another scenario: a lumbar spine MRI might show multiple bulging discs in a patient whose primary issue is actually myofascial back pain—without careful correlation, one might misattribute symptoms to imaging findings. Thus, choosing the test is only half the battle; understanding its results in context is equally crucial.

The table below summarises the *strengths and typical uses* of each modality.

Modality	Key uses	Limitations
X-ray	First-line for bone/joint pathology; fractures, arthritis, calcifications and enthesophytes	Poor soft tissue detail; radiation exposure
Ultrasound	Superficial soft tissues (tendons, bursae, nerves); dynamic assessment; injection guidance; low cost and no radiation	Operator dependent; limited for deep/intraarticular structures
MRI	Best for soft tissue and bone marrow; detects oedema and subtle/occult pathology; complex or red flag cases	Expensive; less available; implant restrictions; incidental findings
CT	Detailed bone and calcifications; fast; useful if MRI contraindicated	Radiation; limited soft tissue detail (unless contrast used)

By aligning the *clinical question* with the modality's strengths, one can efficiently reach a diagnosis while minimising unnecessary tests.

Specific Examples and Imaging Findings in Common Conditions

Tendon Tears

Tendon tears are a frequent concern in soft tissue rheumatology, often arising in the context of chronic tendinopathy or acute injury. Common examples include rotator cuff tears in the shoulder and Achilles tendon tears. Diagnosing a tendon tear accurately is important, as complete tears may require surgical repair, whereas partial tears or tendinosis can often be managed conservatively.

Imaging appearance On *ultrasound*, a full-thickness tendon tear typically appears as an anechoic or hypoechoic defect within the tendon, often with retracted tendon ends and possibly a collection of fluid in the gap. Partial-thickness tears may appear as a focal discontinuity or thinning of fibres, sometimes only visible with dynamic scanning or if the transducer is pressed to show gapping. Ultrasound can also show secondary signs like tendon thickening proximal to the tear (due to tendinopathy) and a *loss of the normal fibrillar pattern* in that region. On *MRI*, tendon tears are best seen on fluid-sensitive sequences, where fluid signals (bright) fill the tear gap. A full-thickness tear of the supraspinatus, for instance, will show fluid extending from the articular to the bursal surface of the tendon, often with tendon retraction and muscle atrophy if chronic. Partial tears may appear as high signal on the bursal or articular side of the tendon without complete discontinuity. In chronic rotator cuff tears, MRI might also demonstrate superior migration of the humeral head or muscle fatty degeneration [17]. Normal tendon on MRI is low signal on all sequences, so a disruption with fluid (high signal) is a clear sign of tearing.

Example—Achilles tendon tear The Achilles is the largest tendon and prone to rupture, especially in middle-aged individuals. Clinically, a complete Achilles rupture is often obvious (with a gap and loss of plantarflexion strength), but partial tears or chronic degenerative tears can be subtle. Ultrasound is useful here: a complete tear shows a gap in the Achilles with frayed edges and hematoma; dynamic ultrasound (Thompson test under the probe) will show no tendon continuity when the calf is squeezed. An *ultrasound image of an Achilles tendon tear* might illustrate a discontinuity in the fibrillar pattern with a hypoechoic fluid-filled gap between the torn ends of the tendon. MRI can also depict Achilles ruptures well, showing the gap and often high-signal oedema in the calf. For Achilles injuries, many clinicians start with ultrasound due to its accessibility; MRI is reserved if the ultrasound is equivocal or if surgical planning demands a more detailed look at adjacent structures (e.g. to assess if the tear extends into the calf muscles).

Accuracy and pitfalls Both ultrasound and MRI are highly accurate for full-thickness tendon tears. Partial tears are more challenging—sensitivity is lower for both modalities (ultrasound may miss small partial tears, and MRI can sometimes under call or overcall partial tears, especially if there is tendinopathy with intrasubstance signal). One pitfall is mistaking tendinosis (which causes tendon thickening and heterogeneity) for a tear. Tendinosis on imaging may show no discrete gap, just diffuse hypoechogenicity on ultrasound or increased tendon signal on MRI without fluid filling a gap. *Clinical correlation* is crucial: not every imaging-detected tear is symptomatic. Many older individuals have asymptomatic rotator cuff tears. Thus, imaging should confirm a suspected tear and correlate with the patient's functional impairment before concluding it is the cause of symptoms.

Bursitis

Bursae are small fluid-filled sacs that reduce friction between tissues (such as where tendons glide over bones). *Bursitis* refers to inflammation of a bursa, often leading to excess fluid accumulation and pain.

Imaging appearance Ultrasound is the imaging modality of choice for evaluating bursitis, as it can directly visualise fluid within a bursa and assess its compressibility and septations. A normal bursa is usually a potential space and not appreciably visible or contains only a trace of fluid. In bursitis, ultrasound will show an *anechoic or hypoechoic fluid collection* in the expected location of the bursa, often with distension of the bursal sac. The bursal walls may appear thickened and hyperaemic if actively inflamed; using power Doppler, one might see increased blood flow in the bursal lining indicating inflammation. For example, in *olecranon bursitis,* an ultrasound reveals a compressible, anechoic fluid pocket over the olecranon process of the ulna, often with some internal echoes if the fluid is complex (as in haemorrhagic or septic bursitis).

Specific Examples

- *Subacromial bursitis* often accompanies rotator cuff tendinopathy or impingement. Ultrasound will show both the bursal fluid and possibly concomitant rotator cuff changes. In chronic impingement, the bursa can become fibrotic and thick—ultrasound then shows a hyperechoic thickened bursal lining.
- *Trochanteric bursitis:* Part of greater trochanteric pain syndrome (which often also involves gluteal tendon tendinopathy). Ultrasound may show fluid in the trochanteric bursa lateral to the hip, though in many cases of trochanteric pain, the bursitis is mild and the main issue is gluteus medius/minimus tendinopathy which ultrasound can also detect. MRI of the hip might show trochanteric bursitis as fluid with surrounding oedema in severe cases.
- *Prepatellar and pes anserine bursitis:* These knee bursae can be visualised on ultrasound as fluid pockets superficial to the patella (prepatellar) or at the pes anserinus (anserine bursa, medially).

Interpreting normal vs pathological Recognising bursitis on imaging often comes down to identifying fluid where normally there is almost none. For example, a *subdeltoid bursa* thickness over 2–3 mm is generally considered abnormal. Research in polymyalgia rheumatica (PMR) has shown that bilateral subacromial-subdeltoid bursitis detected on ultrasound is a distinguishing feature of PMR and rarely seen in simple degenerative shoulder disease [18]. Normal individuals might have a thin <1 mm bursal line, whereas pathological bursae are distended and sometimes multiloculated [19].

Clinical correlation and urgency Most bursitis cases are benign and managed conservatively, but a key consideration is *septic bursitis*. If the clinical scenario suggests infection (e.g. olecranon bursitis with erythema, warmth, systemic fever), imaging can help by confirming fluid is present, but the definitive step is aspiration. Ultrasound can guide a needle into the bursa for diagnostic fluid aspiration and analysis. In an instance where septic bursitis is suspected but the bursal fluid cannot be easily aspirated (perhaps due to very thick fluid or difficult access), an MRI may be warranted to evaluate for adjacent abscess formation or cellulitis tracking and to locate fluid for a possible drainage [20].

Calcific Tendinitis

Calcific tendinitis is a condition where calcium hydroxyapatite crystals deposit in tendons or peritendinous structures, most commonly around the shoulder (rotator cuff tendons) but also in other areas like the gluteal tendons, Achilles tendon or wrist. The shoulder form—often termed *calcific tendinopathy of the rotator cuff*—is a classic cause of acute or chronic shoulder pain, typically in middle age. These deposits can cause pain by creating inflammation in the tendon or adjacent bursa (especially during the resorptive phase when the calcium can extrude and incite bursitis).

Imaging appearance Plain *X-ray is the simplest first test* for calcific tendinitis in superficial locations like the shoulder. The calcium deposits appear as homogeneous, amorphous dense opacities in the soft tissues near the tendon insertion. In the shoulder, they are usually in the supraspinatus tendon region, just distal to its attachment on the greater tubercle. They may be round or oval "chalky" looking deposits, often 1–2 cm in size, but can be fragmented or multiple. X-rays should be done in at least two views (e.g. internal and external rotation views of the shoulder) because calcifications can be obscured by bone in certain projections. Fig. 3.1 shows a shoulder X-ray with calcific tendinitis: note the globular opaque calcium deposit in the rotator cuff area (supraspinatus tendon), distinct from the bone.

On *ultrasound*, calcific deposits are highly echogenic foci within the tendon, usually with acoustic shadowing (especially if the deposit is dense and well-formed) [21]. Ultrasound can not only detect the calcium but also assess its consistency (hard and unyielding vs mushy), which is important because more "cystic" or gelatinous calcium deposits indicate the resorptive phase and might be amenable to aspiration with a needle. Ultrasound has the advantage of being able to guide *percutaneous needle lavage* of calcific tendinitis—a procedure where the deposit is needled and washed out under local anaesthesia. Additionally, ultrasound can evaluate the rotator cuff integrity around the calcification (some patients with calcific tendinitis also have coexisting tendon tears or tendinosis) [21].

MRI is *not the first-line modality* for calcific tendinitis because the calcium deposits can appear as nonspecific low-signal areas that might be missed if small [22]. On MRI, a calcium deposit usually shows as a dark signal on both T1 and T2 (since calcium is low signal intensity), and there may be surrounding oedema or bursitis that is high signal. MRI may be done if the diagnosis is unclear or if there is suspicion of another problem alongside the calcific tendinitis (e.g., to check if there is a rotator cuff tear under the calcification, as very large calcium deposits can sometimes cause tendon rupture). Generally, *X-ray combined with ultrasound* gives the most information for calcific tendinitis, and MRI/CT are reserved for atypical cases or if initial treatments fail and surgery is contemplated.

Clinical correlation Calcific tendinitis can be very painful, especially when the calcium is releasing into the bursa (causing an acute bursitis often called "calcific bursitis"). On imaging, that scenario might show the deposit breaking up and fluid in the bursa. The correlation between imaging and symptoms can sometimes be surprising—some patients have large deposits on X-ray and minimal pain (especially if the deposits are in a chronic phase), whereas others have small deposits that are exquisitely painful when acutely inflamed. The presence of *bursal fluid and hypervascularity on Doppler* tends to correlate with acute pain [23]. During this phase, an intervention (like ultrasound-guided needling or a steroid injection into

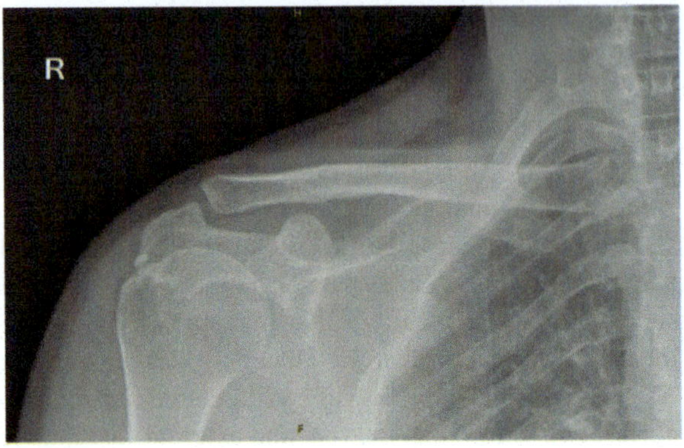

Fig. 3.1 X-ray of a right shoulder demonstrating a globular calcific tendinitis deposit in the supraspinatus tendon

the bursa) could dramatically relieve symptoms by evacuating the calcium and reducing inflammation.

Management implications Imaging not only diagnoses calcific tendinitis but can guide treatment. A large, well-formed calcification visible on X-ray can be targeted by ultrasound-guided lavage. If repeated nonsurgical measures fail, surgical removal of the deposit may be considered—in such cases, the exact location and size of the deposit as shown on imaging help the surgeon plan the approach (some deposits are actually intramuscular or intratendinous and need careful localisation). The good news is that many calcific deposits eventually dissolve on their own, which can be monitored on serial X-rays—one might see a calcific deposit gradually shrinking or disappearing over months, often corresponding to resolution of symptoms.

Enthesopathies (Enthesitis)

Enthesopathy refers to disorders of the enthesis—the site where tendons or ligaments insert into bone. When these insertions are inflamed, it is called *enthesitis* [24]. Enthesitis is a hallmark of the spondyloarthropathies (SpA), but enthesopathy can also occur from mechanical stress (e.g. a heel spur at the Achilles insertion from chronic traction). Common sites include the Achilles tendon insertion on the calcaneus, the plantar fascia origin on the calcaneus, patellar tendon insertions on the patella and tibial tubercle and the epicondyles of the elbow (common flexor and extensor origins).

Imaging appearance Entheses can be evaluated by multiple modalities, each revealing different aspects:

- *Ultrasound:* Musculoskeletal ultrasound has emerged as a sensitive tool for detecting enthesitis [25]. Ultrasound can directly visualise the enthesis, showing features of active inflammation such as *increased thickness* of the tendon or ligament at the insertion, *hypoechogenicity* (indicating oedema) and *power Doppler signal* indicating active blood flow/inflammation at the enthesis. It can also show structural damage like *erosions* at the bone attachment or *enthesophytes* (bony spurs). For example, in an Achilles enthesitis (as seen in spondyloarthritis), ultrasound might show a thickened Achilles tendon near its calcaneal insertion with loss of the normal fibrillar pattern, perhaps small erosions in the calcaneus at the insertion point, calcifications within the tendon and Doppler signal if the enthesis is actively inflamed.

- *X-ray:* Conventional radiographs mainly show the *chronic changes* of enthesopathy, such as enthesophytes (calcific bone spurs) or gross calcification of attachments. For instance, a large inferior calcaneal spur on X-ray is a sign of chronic plantar fasciitis enthesopathy.
- *MRI:* MRI can detect *early enthesitis changes* that X-rays cannot. Particularly, MRI will show bone marrow oedema at the enthesis (in the adjacent bone) as a hallmark of active enthesitis in spondyloarthritis [26]. For example, an MRI of the heel in reactive arthritis might show bone marrow oedema in the calcaneus where the Achilles attaches, along with high signal in the tendon insertion itself and maybe swelling of the retrocalcaneal bursa if coinvolved. MRI also can depict the erosions or proliferative changes at entheses and any associated soft tissue oedema. Whole-body MRI is a research tool that can screen many entheses at once for inflammation in SpA. However, MRI is not as readily used for enthesitis in routine practice unless there is a specific diagnostic dilemma, given the cost and need to image multiple sites potentially.
- *CT:* CT has a limited role except to better delineate the bony spurs or erosions if needed. It could show, for example, a very fine enthesophyte that an X-ray might miss. CT is generally unnecessary for enthesitis except perhaps in axial disease (like evaluating a sacroiliac joint fusion or spinal ligament calcification), which goes beyond soft tissue into axial skeletal imaging.

Normal versus pathological enthesis Normally, an enthesis may have a little irregularity at the bone attachment, especially in older patients or those with a history of stress. Some small spurs can even be seen in asymptomatic people (like a mild heel spur). What denotes pathology is typically a combination of changes: *thickening of the tendon/ligament at insertion, erosive changes in bone, calcifications and Doppler signal indicating inflammation*. In active spondyloarthropathy, multiple entheses might show such changes simultaneously. It is noteworthy that *enthesitis can also cause adjacent bursitis* (e.g. retrocalcaneal bursitis may coexist with insertional Achilles tendinopathy, particularly in the setting of a posterosuperior calcaneal prominence, as seen in Haglund syndrome). Ultrasound might show fluid in the bursa along with the tendon changes.

In terms of diagnosis, the *Outcome Measures in Rheumatology (OMERACT)* group has developed definitions for ultrasound enthesitis, including criteria like hypoechogenicity, thickening, enthesophytes and Doppler signal at enthesis [27]. Adhering to such criteria improves the reliability of ultrasound as a diagnostic tool for enthesitis.

Red Flags: When Urgent Imaging Is Required

While most soft tissue rheumatologic conditions are benign and subacute, it is crucial to stay vigilant for *red flag signs* that may indicate a more serious underlying pathology requiring urgent imaging or intervention. These red flags might emerge from the history or physical exam and should prompt immediate further investigation rather than the usual conservative approach. Key red flags include the following:

- *Severe unremitting pain, especially night pain or systemic symptoms:* If a patient with what seems like a soft tissue complaint reports *night pain that wakes them, unexplained weight loss or fevers,* one must consider possibilities like infection or tumour. For example, constant bone-deep pain not relieved by rest could signal an occult bone malignancy or infection rather than a simple tendinopathy. In such cases, advanced imaging (MRI) is warranted quickly. A classic teaching is that *night pain and weight loss are red flags for malignancy* in musculoskeletal presentations [28]. Depending on the clinical context, this may require plain radiographs and/or targeted cross-sectional imaging, such as MRI for suspected local musculoskeletal malignancy or CT chest if a Pancoast tumour is suspected.
- *Erythema, warmth or signs of infection in a focal area:* If a patient has a red, hot, swollen structure (e.g. an olecranon bursa that is very red and tender), think septic bursitis or even necrotising infection. *Immediate aspiration* (which is a diagnostic procedure rather than imaging) is indicated for suspected septic bursitis or septic arthritis. But imaging like ultrasound can assist by confirming fluid and guiding the needle. If aspiration cannot be done or the area is worsening, urgent MRI can help delineate an abscess or extent of infection. In necrotising fasciitis (a medical emergency), plain X-ray or CT might show subcutaneous gas, which is a surgical emergency sign. Essentially, *infection—do not delay imaging or referral.* Another example is suspected spinal infection (discitis or abscess) in a patient with back pain and fever—that is a red flag requiring urgent MRI of the spine.
- *History of significant trauma or acute functional loss:* If a patient felt a "pop" in the knee and cannot extend it, one must suspect a tendon rupture (like quadriceps or patellar tendon rupture). Similarly, inability to plantarflex the ankle after an injury points to an Achilles tendon rupture. These situations require immediate imaging confirmation if the clinical exam is equivocal, because early surgical repair may be needed. An X-ray could show an avulsion fragment (e.g. patella alta on X-ray for patellar tendon rupture), and an ultrasound or MRI can quickly confirm the tear.
- *Possible cauda equina syndrome or cord compression:* Though this strays into spine territory, rheumatologists do encounter neck/back issues. *Red flags like new limb weakness, bowel/bladder dysfunction and saddle anaesthesia* require immediate MRI to look for cord compression (from a large disc, hematoma, etc.) [29]. Even though this might not be a typical "soft tissue rheumatology" scenario, it is a crucial red flag scenario that demands urgent imaging and often surgical evaluation.

- *Unusual swelling or mass in soft tissue:* Most localised swellings rheumatologists see are benign (ganglia, lipomas, Baker's cysts, etc.), but a firm growing mass, especially if deep, is a red flag for possible sarcoma. In such cases, rather than repeated ultrasounds or aspirations, one should obtain appropriate imaging (MRI is the modality of choice for characterising a soft tissue mass) and refer to orthopaedics/oncology. Imaging can differentiate cystic from solid masses and help in biopsy planning. For instance, what is presumed to be "chronic bursitis" over the knee that is not responding to therapy and feels unusually firm should be imaged to ensure it is not a synovial sarcoma or pigmented villonodular synovitis (PVNS).
- *Multiple sites of pain with systemic features:* If a patient presents with many tender entheses and also has fever or weight loss, one might worry about something like diffuse idiopathic skeletal hyperostosis (DISH) or metastatic cancer affecting multiple sites. While blood tests (like inflammatory markers) would also be done, imaging might include a bone scan or PET scan to screen for multifocal pathology. This is rare but worth noting: for example, multiple "tendonitis" sites plus high alkaline phosphatase might make one consider imaging for hypertrophic osteoarthropathy or metastases.

In summary, *urgent imaging is required when red flags suggest infection, malignancy, acute neurovascular compromise or serious injury*. In these scenarios, the threshold for imaging is low, and the modality is chosen based on what will best reveal the suspected issue (often MRI for soft tissue/cord, CT for detailed bone or when MRI is not possible and radiographs for initial trauma survey). Clinicians should maintain a high index of suspicion and promptly escalate to appropriate imaging and specialty referral when these red flags are present.

Laboratory Investigations in Soft Tissue Rheumatology

While imaging is critical, laboratory tests play a complementary role in diagnosing soft tissue rheumatologic conditions, especially for distinguishing *noninflammatory vs inflammatory* aetiologies and identifying systemic diseases that might manifest with soft tissue pain. Not every patient with a tendon or bursa issue needs blood tests—in many isolated mechanical problems (like tennis elbow or trochanteric bursitis in an otherwise healthy person), bloods are usually normal. However, in the right clinical context, labs can confirm a suspected rheumatic disease or reveal an unexpected diagnosis. Key laboratory investigations include the following:

- *Acute phase reactants (ESR and CRP):* The erythrocyte sedimentation rate (ESR) and C-reactive protein (CRP) are general markers of inflammation. In purely mechanical soft tissue conditions, these markers are usually normal. If you find a significantly elevated ESR/CRP in a patient with a presumed soft tissue pathology, it should raise suspicion of an underlying *inflammatory or infectious process*. For example, a patient with bilateral shoulder and hip pain and stiffness has an ESR of 80 mm/hr—this strongly supports polymyalgia rheumatica over a mechanical cause, especially if imaging (ultrasound) shows bilateral subdeltoid bursitis, as studies have shown this combination is highly characteristic for PMR [18]. Acute phase reactants are also invaluable in monitoring or identifying *infection*: for instance, if septic bursitis is suspected, CRP is often elevated and can be trended to see if treatment is effective. In septic arthritis, the combination of fever, high CRP/ESR is a red flag that should prompt joint aspiration.

- *Autoantibodies and immune markers:* In patients where an underlying autoimmune rheumatic disease is suspected, tests such as rheumatoid factor (RF), anti-citrullinated protein antibody (anti-CCP), antinuclear antibody (ANA) or others (SSA, SSB, etc.) might be appropriate. For example, consider a patient with chronic Achilles tendon pain and swelling in the context of a wider picture like inflammatory back pain and some finger swelling—one might test HLA-B27 (a genetic marker associated with spondyloarthropathies) [30]. Or if a patient has bilateral wrist tenosynovitis and a couple of swollen finger joints, checking RF and anti-CCP could confirm rheumatoid arthritis as the cause of their tendon issues. Often, *tenosynovitis* in hands or feet is an early sign of rheumatoid arthritis, and positive serologies would clinch the diagnosis. Similarly, *ANA* and other antibodies might be checked if one suspects a connective tissue disease (though these classically cause more articular or systemic issues, sometimes they can present with soft tissue manifestations, like myositis causing muscle tenderness or lupus causing tendon laxity). One should note that these tests are not indicated for a routine isolated enthesopathy or bursitis unless there are other clues—for instance, it is not necessary to check ANA/RF in a healthy young patient with the tennis elbow. But if that patient also had other joint symptoms or systemic features, then testing would be broadened.
- *Muscle enzymes:* In cases where muscle pain or weakness is in the differential (e.g. one is considering polymyositis vs a soft tissue shoulder pain), lab tests like creatine kinase (CK) or aldolase can be informative. For example, a patient thought to have trochanteric bursitis but who actually has difficulty climbing stairs due to muscle weakness might need CK tested to evaluate for myositis.
- *Metabolic and crystal-related tests:* Soft tissue rheumatology overlaps with metabolic conditions at times. *Serum uric acid* is a relevant test if gout is in the differential. Although gout typically causes joint arthritis, it can present as bursitis (e.g. olecranon bursitis due to gouty tophi) or tendinous tophi (urate crystals depositing in tendons can cause a chronic tendinopathy). If an olecranon bursal aspirate reveals monosodium urate crystals, that confirms gouty bursitis. Checking serum urate helps in the long-term management of gout. *Calcium pyrophosphate* deposition (pseudogout) can also affect tendons and bursae (for instance, calcific deposition in the ligamentum flavum, Achilles, etc.), though crystal diagnosis is usually by aspiration and microscopy rather than blood tests. *Calcium and phosphate levels* might be checked if one suspects tumoural calcinosis or metabolic causes of calcification, but that is rare. One metabolic condition worth noting is hyperparathyroidism—it can cause tendon calcifications and

bone resorption [31]. If one saw multiple tendon calcifications on X-ray in an atypical distribution, checking calcium/PTH could be indicated.

- *Synovial fluid analysis:* While not a blood test, analysing fluid from a bursa or tendon sheath is a laboratory investigation of great importance. If a bursa is aspirated, the fluid can be sent for *cell count, Gram stain/culture and crystal analysis*. Aspiration and analysis is the gold standard for differentiating infectious vs crystal vs inflammatory bursitis and should be performed whenever those diagnoses are in question.
- *Specific rheumatic disease markers:* In certain contexts, additional tests may be done. For example, if *vasculitis* involving peritendinous structures is considered, one might check ANCA (antineutrophil cytoplasmic antibodies) [32]. In a patient with diffuse pain and fatigue where fibromyalgia vs something like hypothyroidism is debated, a TSH test (thyroid-stimulating hormone) is a relevant test (hypothyroidism can cause myalgias and even carpal tunnel syndrome) [33]. Vitamin D levels might be checked in diffuse pain syndromes (though evidence of direct correlation is mild, repleting low vitamin D is generally advisable).

When and why to order blood tests The decision to order labs in a soft tissue rheumatology evaluation is driven by suspicion of *systemic disease or atypical features.* Generally:

- If the presentation is *focal and mechanical-appearing* (e.g. unilateral tennis elbow in a tennis player, otherwise healthy), extensive lab testing is low yield and not necessary.
- If there are *multiple sites of musculoskeletal pain, constitutional symptoms or chronicity beyond what is expected,* labs are indicated to rule out systemic rheumatic diseases. For instance, someone with bilateral Achilles tendinopathies, plantar fasciitis and low back stiffness should get HLA-B27 and inflammatory markers to assess for a spondyloarthropathy.
- If initial treatment fails or the condition relapses unusually, consider labs, for example, a presumed trochanteric bursitis that keeps recurring despite steroid injections—perhaps check ANA or rheumatoid factor to see if an underlying RA or lupus is present that causes chronic periarthritis.
- *Baseline labs before therapy:* Sometimes bloods are done not to diagnose but to ensure safety before treatments. For example, if considering a corticosteroid injection, one might check blood glucose in diabetics (as steroids can spike it). Or before starting an NSAID regularly, some clinicians check kidney function or blood pressure, though those are more management considerations than diagnostic.

It is also worth noting that *blood tests can be normal in many soft tissue rheumatic conditions.* Normal ESR/CRP does not entirely exclude an inflammatory condition, but it makes it less likely (e.g. a small percentage of polymyalgia rheumatica patients can have normal ESR—in such cases, imaging like ultrasound may carry more weight). Likewise, seronegative rheumatoid arthritis is a possibility (RF and CCP negative), so negative serologies do not completely rule out RA if clinical picture is convincing, but they lower the probability.

In summary, *laboratory investigations are used selectively* in soft tissue rheumatology: to confirm suspected systemic diseases (inflammatory markers, autoantibodies), to identify crystal arthropathies (fluid analysis, urate levels) and to ensure we are not missing an infection (FBC, CRP, culture of aspirate). The integration of lab results with imaging findings and clinical assessment forms a comprehensive diagnostic approach. For instance, if a patient has a high CRP and ultrasound evidence of bilateral bursitis and tenosynovitis, we lean towards a systemic inflammatory rheumatism (like PMR or RA) and treat accordingly. If bloods are normal and imaging shows only localised changes, a local therapy and biomechanical approach are favoured.

Diagnostic Algorithm: Integrating Clinical Assessment, Imaging and Labs

The evaluation of a patient with a soft tissue musculoskeletal complaint can be approached stepwise, integrating clinical findings with judicious use of imaging and lab tests.

The *initial clinical assessment* (history and physical exam, as described in Chap. 2) guides the next steps:

1. *Mechanical vs inflammatory clues:* Determine if the presentation is more suggestive of a local mechanical lesion or if there are signs of systemic or inflammatory disease. Key questions: Is the pain isolated to one site or multiple? Are there swelling, warmth, morning stiffness >30 minutes (inflammatory) or just activity-related pain (mechanical)? Are there constitutional symptoms like fever or fatigue?
2. *Red flags present?* If any red flags (severe pain at rest/night, weight loss, fever, neurodeficits, acute trauma with deformity) are present, do not delay—proceed to *urgent imaging or intervention*. For example, if suspect infection, aspirate and consider emergent MRI; if suspect fracture or major tear, get immediate X-ray, ultrasound, etc. Red flags generally bypass conservative trial—*immediate diagnostic imaging and referral* is warranted.
3. *Initial Imaging—X-ray if indicated:* In many cases (especially older patients or after trauma), an X-ray is a prudent first imaging to look for obvious bony pathology or calcifications. If the X-ray yields a diagnosis (e.g. shows calcific tendinitis, osteoarthritis or a fracture), you might manage based on that and only do further imaging if needed for treatment planning. If X-ray is normal or not done (for instance, in a young patient with a classic tendinopathy and no red flags, you might skip straight to ultrasound), proceed accordingly.

4. *Ultrasound vs MRI decision:* This is the crux for most soft tissue diagnoses:

   - If the structure of interest is *accessible to ultrasound* (e.g. peripheral tendon, bursa, superficial joint) and the question is focused (tear vs no tear, fluid vs no fluid), ultrasound is often the next step. It is especially favoured if real-time examination or guided injection might be done in the same session.
   - If the area is *deep or complex* (e.g. hip joint or spine) or if multiple tissue types need evaluation (bone marrow, cartilage, etc.) or if ultrasound is not readily available/expertly performed, then *MRI is indicated.*
   - If ultrasound results are equivocal or incomplete, and clinical suspicion remains, escalate to MRI.
   - For certain diagnoses like suspected nerve compression or muscle injury, MRI may be better (though ultrasound can see peripheral nerves to a degree as well).

5. *Blood tests in parallel:* If initial clinical impression and imaging suggest a purely local mechanical issue, extensive labs may not be necessary. However, if there are *any systemic features or multiple sites*, order appropriate labs in parallel with imaging. For example, if an ultrasound of a hand shows tenosynovitis in multiple flexor tendons, check RF/anti-CCP to assess for RA. Labs can sometimes be the clue that triggers reconsideration of the diagnosis (e.g. a high CRP in "tendonitis" prompting a closer look for infection or rheumatic disease). Conversely, completely normal labs can reinforce that a condition is likely localised (though as noted, not all inflammation elevates bloods).
6. *Synthesis and differential diagnosis:* Once imaging and lab results are in, integrate them. There are a few branching outcomes:

   - *Clear diagnosis achieved:* For example, ultrasound shows lateral epicondylitis with no tear; labs are normal—diagnosis is tennis elbow (degenerative tendinopathy). Or MRI shows partial rotator cuff tear and subacromial bursitis, with mild CRP elevation—likely impingement plus some inflammation but not a systemic disease. Manage accordingly (physiotherapy, injections, etc., as discussed in later chapters).
   - *Inconclusive results:* If imaging is negative or nonspecific and labs are normal, consider that the issue might be nonstructural (e.g. referred pain, fibromyalgia if widespread tenderness with normal tests, etc.). Reassess the patient: is the pain out of proportion to findings? This might be when to consider other diagnoses or a trial of therapy with close follow-up rather than more tests.
   - *Discrepant findings:* Sometimes imaging might show one thing and labs suggest another. For example, mild tendon tear on ultrasound but labs show high inflammatory markers and positive rheumatoid factor. This could mean the patient has rheumatoid arthritis causing tenosynovitis on top of a degenerative tear. In such cases, you would need to address both: treat the underlying RA (with systemic therapy) and the local tendon issue as needed. Always

explain discrepancies by considering a unifying diagnosis or coexisting conditions.

- *Need for additional tests:* If after first-line imaging and basic labs the diagnosis remains unclear, consider second-line investigations. These could include *advanced imaging* (CT, bone scan, PET if tumour/infection in question), *specialised tests* (e.g. muscle biopsy or genetic tests in unusual myopathies) or *referral for tissue biopsy* (if imaging finds a mass or atypical lesion).

7. *Reevaluation:* The diagnostic process is iterative. If initial treatments are implemented (assuming a working diagnosis) but the patient does not improve as expected, revisit the diagnostic algorithm. Something might have been missed—maybe the patient labelled with "chronic bursitis" actually has an underlying psoriatic arthritis causing repeated enthesitis. In such a scenario, one might reorder labs (like checking psoriasis history and doing an ultrasound which shows power Doppler enthesitis rather than simple bursitis).

This method underscores a core principle: *start broad by ruling out dangerous or systemic causes (red flags, labs for inflammation) and then focus on confirming the local diagnosis with targeted imaging, and finally correlate everything to ensure it fits together.* It is about being neither overreliant on imaging nor on labs but using both as needed to arrive at the correct diagnosis that explains the patient's symptoms.

By following a structured approach and knowing when to deploy each diagnostic tool, clinicians can efficiently navigate even complex soft tissue rheumatologic cases. The end result should be a clear diagnosis (or a short differential) that will inform effective management—which is the focus of later chapters.

Key Learning Points

- *Imaging as extension of exam:* In soft tissue rheumatology, imaging (ultrasound, MRI, X-ray, CT) serves to confirm clinical suspicions, assess the extent of injuries and occasionally reveal alternative diagnoses. It should be used purposefully—answer a specific clinical question with the most appropriate modality rather than "imaging everything".
- *Ultrasound first for many soft tissue lesions:* Ultrasound offers real-time, high-resolution evaluation of tendons, bursae and entheses without radiation. It has diagnostic accuracy comparable to MRI for many tendon tears [5], and it additionally permits dynamic assessment and guided injections. Operator skill is critical for optimal results. Use ultrasound especially for superficial structures and guided aspirations/injections.
- *MRI for deep or complex cases:* MRI provides comprehensive views of soft tissue and bone marrow and is indispensable for detecting occult pathology (e.g. bone oedema in enthesitis, muscle tears or tumours). Reserve MRI for when ultrasound is insufficient—such as deep joint pain and unexplained symptoms

with normal X-ray/US—or when red flags suggest serious pathology needing detailed evaluation.

- *X-rays are still valuable:* Always consider a plain radiograph in the initial work-up, particularly to check for fractures, degenerative changes or calcifications. A simple X-ray can diagnose calcific tendinitis or reveal an unexpected bone lesion. Remember that a normal X-ray does not rule out soft tissue injury, but an abnormal X-ray can significantly alter the diagnostic pathway.
- *Strengths and limits of each modality: Ultrasound*—great for soft tissues, no radiation, but user-dependent and limited depth. *MRI*—excellent detail and sensitivity for inflammation but expensive and slower. *CT*—best for bone detail and calcifications but high radiation and limited soft tissue info. *X-ray*— fast screening for bone/calcific changes but poor for soft tissue detail. Knowing these helps in test selection.
- *Interpretation—normal vs pathologic:* Learn the imaging appearance of normal tendons, bursae, etc., to recognise pathology. For example, normal tendons are continuous and fibrillar; a tear shows discontinuity. Normal bursae are virtual; bursitis shows fluid distension. Normal enthesis may have a small spur in older age; active enthesitis shows thickening, erosions and Doppler signal. Distinguish incidental age-related changes from acute pathology by correlation with symptoms and inflammatory signs.
- *Red flags require urgency:* Signs like fever with joint/bursa swelling, unrelenting night pain, acute muscle weakness or history of cancer in a musculoskeletal pain patient mandate prompt imaging and possibly referral. These scenarios aim to exclude infection, malignancy or severe injuries (like tendon ruptures or spinal compression) and should not be managed with watchful waiting.
- *Laboratory tests complement imaging:* Consider using ESR/CRP to gauge inflammation—high values can signal polymyalgia rheumatica, rheumatoid arthritis or infection rather than a simple strain. Autoantibodies (RF, CCP, ANA) help confirm underlying rheumatic diseases when clinical clues exist (e.g. tenosynovitis or multiple enthesitis). Always analyse any accessible fluid (bursal or joint aspirate) for crystals and infection if septic or crystal arthritis is in the differential. Normal labs generally point towards localised/mechanical aetiologies, whereas abnormal labs push towards systemic/inflammatory diagnoses.
- *Integrated diagnostic approach:* The best practice is integrating clinical evaluation with targeted investigations. A diagnostic system can guide clinicians: assess clinical pattern → rule out red flags → start with basic imaging (X-ray) if indicated → proceed to ultrasound or MRI based on needs → order labs if inflammatory or systemic disease suspected → synthesise all information. This approach maximises diagnostic yield and minimises unnecessary procedures.
- *Case application:* Returning to the case vignette—the patient with recalcitrant "tennis elbow" and slight olecranon swelling—following these principles: an ultrasound could be done to differentiate tendon vs bursal pathology; an X-ray might be ordered to look for calcification or arthritis if trauma or spurs are a concern; and given atypical features (effusion, warmth), an inflammatory marker test (CRP) could be checked. Suppose ultrasound reveals extensor tendinosis *and*

an olecranon bursitis with crystal deposits and lab shows high uric acid—we might discover gouty bursitis contributing to the picture, changing management. This underscores how a careful mix of imaging and lab investigations can uncover the true diagnosis and direct appropriate therapy.

With a systematic use of diagnostic tools, clinicians can approach soft tissue rheumatology cases with confidence, ensuring that underlying causes are correctly identified and that patients receive timely, effective treatment based on accurate diagnoses.

References

1. Tins BJ, Butler R. Imaging in rheumatology: reconciling radiology and rheumatology. Insights Imaging [Internet]. 2013;4(6):799–810. Available from: http://www.ncbi.nlm.nih.gov/pubmed/24127271
2. Endara-Mina J, Kumar H, Ghosh B, Mehta A, Chandra Dey R, Singh P, et al. Comparative use of ultrasound and radiography for the detection of fractures: a systematic review and narrative synthesis. Ann Med Surg [Internet]. 2023;85(10):5085–95. Available from: http://www.ncbi.nlm.nih.gov/pubmed/37811018
3. Grassi W, Salaffi F, Filippucci E. Ultrasound in rheumatology. Best Pract Res Clin Rheumatol [Internet]. 2005;19(3):467–85. Available from: http://www.ncbi.nlm.nih.gov/pubmed/15939370
4. Carotti M, Galeazzi V, Catucci F, Zappia M, Arrigoni F, Barile A, et al. Clinical utility of eco-color-power Doppler ultrasonography and contrast enhanced magnetic resonance imaging for interpretation and quantification of joint synovitis: a review. Acta Biomed [Internet]. 2018;89(1-S):48–77. Available from: http://www.ncbi.nlm.nih.gov/pubmed/29350637
5. Roy J-S, Braën C, Leblond J, Desmeules F, Dionne CE, MacDermid JC, et al. Diagnostic accuracy of ultrasonography, MRI and MR arthrography in the characterisation of rotator cuff disorders: a systematic review and meta-analysis. Br J Sports Med [Internet]. 2015;49(20):1316–28. Available from: http://www.ncbi.nlm.nih.gov/pubmed/25677796
6. Toh Y. Ultrasound versus magnetic resonance imaging as first-line imaging strategies for rotator cuff pathologies: a comprehensive analysis of clinical practices, economic efficiency, and future perspectives. Cureus [Internet]. 2024;16(4):e59231. Available from: http://www.ncbi.nlm.nih.gov/pubmed/38813323
7. Ohrndorf S, Naumann L, Grundey J, Scheel T, Scheel AK, Werner C, et al. Is musculoskeletal ultrasonography an operator-dependent method or a fast and reliably teachable diagnostic tool? Interreader agreements of three ultrasonographers with different training levels. Int J Rheumatol [Internet]. 2010;2010:164518. Available from: http://www.ncbi.nlm.nih.gov/pubmed/21197088
8. Bianchi S. Ultrasound and bone: a pictorial review. J Ultrasound [Internet]. 2020;23(3):227–57. Available from: http://www.ncbi.nlm.nih.gov/pubmed/32419074
9. Eustace S, Keogh C, Blake M, Ward RJ, Oder PD, Dimasi M. MR imaging of bone oedema: mechanisms and interpretation. Clin Radiol [Internet]. 2001;56(1):4–12. Available from: http://www.ncbi.nlm.nih.gov/pubmed/11162690
10. Bakewell C, Aydin SZ, Ranganath VK, Eder L, Kaeley GS. Imaging techniques: options for the diagnosis and monitoring of treatment of enthesitis in psoriatic arthritis. J Rheumatol [Internet]. 2020;47(7):973–82. Available from: http://www.jrheum.org/lookup/doi/10.3899/jrheum.190512
11. Ghadimi M, Thomas A. Magnetic resonance imaging contraindications [Internet]. In: StatPearls; 2026. Available from: http://www.ncbi.nlm.nih.gov/pubmed/15556662.

12. Dereli Bulut SS, Akcayoz B, Candan ES, Sakci Z, Soylemez MS. Deciphering pain through imaging: what do MRI and ultrasound reveal in calcific tendinopathy? Skeletal Radiol [Internet]. 2026;55(1):223–30. Available from: http://www.ncbi.nlm.nih.gov/pubmed/40824328
13. Carrino JA, Ibad H, Lin Y, Ghotbi E, Klein J, Demehri S, et al. CT in musculoskeletal imaging: still helpful and for what? Skeletal Radiol [Internet]. 2024;53(9):1711–25. Available from: http://www.ncbi.nlm.nih.gov/pubmed/38969781
14. Fred HL. Drawbacks and limitations of computed tomography: views from a medical educator. Texas Hear Inst J [Internet]. 2004;31(4):345–8. Available from: http://www.ncbi.nlm.nih.gov/pubmed/15745283
15. Ory PA. Radiography in the assessment of musculoskeletal conditions. Best Pract Res Clin Rheumatol [Internet]. 2003;17(3):495–512. Available from: http://www.ncbi.nlm.nih.gov/pubmed/12787514
16. Vijayanathan S, Butt S, Gnanasegaran G, Groves AM. Advantages and limitations of imaging the musculoskeletal system by conventional radiological, radionuclide, and hybrid modalities. Semin Nucl Med [Internet]. 2009;39(6):357–68. Available from: http://www.ncbi.nlm.nih.gov/pubmed/19801216
17. Siow MY, Mitchell BC, Hachadorian M, Wang W, Bastrom T, Kent WT, et al. Association between rotator cuff tears and superior migration of the humeral head: an MRI-based anatomic study. Orthop J Sport Med [Internet]. 2021;9(6):23259671211009850. Available from: http://www.ncbi.nlm.nih.gov/pubmed/34179206
18. Terenzi R, Ditto MC, Benucci M, Mannoni A, Guiducci S, Fusaro E, et al. Ultrasound-detected bilateral subacromial-subdeltoid bursitis exceeding 3 mm differentiates polymyalgia rheumatica from rotator cuff tendinopathy: a cross-sectional observational study. Rheumatol Int [Internet]. 2025;45(9):216. Available from: http://www.ncbi.nlm.nih.gov/pubmed/40892101
19. Couanis G, Breidahl W, Burnham S. The relationship between subacromial bursa thickness on ultrasound and shoulder pain in open water endurance swimmers over time. J Sci Med Sport [Internet]. 2015;18(4):373–7. Available from: http://www.ncbi.nlm.nih.gov/pubmed/24907190
20. Truong J, Mabrouk A, Ashurst JV. Septic bursitis [Internet]. In: StatPearls; 2026. Available from: http://www.ncbi.nlm.nih.gov/pubmed/30479679.
21. Chianca V, Albano D, Messina C, Midiri F, Mauri G, Aliprandi A, et al. Rotator cuff calcific tendinopathy: from diagnosis to treatment. Acta Biomed [Internet]. 2018;89(1-S):186–96. Available from: http://www.ncbi.nlm.nih.gov/pubmed/29350647
22. Merolla G, Bhat MG, Paladini P, Porcellini G. Complications of calcific tendinitis of the shoulder: a concise review. J Orthop Traumatol [Internet]. 2015;16(3):175–83. Available from: http://www.ncbi.nlm.nih.gov/pubmed/25697847
23. Inoue A, Funakoshi T, Koga R, Kusano H, Takahashi T, Miyamoto A, et al. Evaluation of hypervascularity in synovitis of the shoulder using ultrasound: comparison of preoperative ultrasound findings and intraoperative arthroscopic findings. JSES Int [Internet]. 2022;6(3):473–8. Available from: http://www.ncbi.nlm.nih.gov/pubmed/35572442
24. Sudoł-Szopińska I, Kwiatkowska B, Prochorec-Sobieszek M, Maśliński W. Enthesopathies and enthesitis. Part 1. Etiopathogenesis. J Ultrason [Internet]. 2015;15(60):72–84. Available from: http://www.ncbi.nlm.nih.gov/pubmed/26674568
25. Gandjbakhch F, Terslev L, Joshua F, Wakefield RJ, Naredo E, D'Agostino MA, et al. Ultrasound in the evaluation of enthesitis: status and perspectives. Arthritis Res Ther [Internet]. 2011;13(6):R188. Available from: http://www.ncbi.nlm.nih.gov/pubmed/22093457
26. Eshed I, Bollow M, McGonagle DG, Tan AL, Althoff CE, Asbach P, et al. MRI of enthesitis of the appendicular skeleton in spondyloarthritis. Ann Rheum Dis [Internet]. 2007;66(12):1553–9. Available from: http://www.ncbi.nlm.nih.gov/pubmed/17526551
27. Filippucci E, Smerilli G, Di Matteo A, Grassi W. Ultrasound definition of enthesitis in spondyloarthritis and psoriatic arthritis: arrival or starting point? Ann Rheum Dis [Internet]. 2021;80(11):1373–5. Available from: http://www.ncbi.nlm.nih.gov/pubmed/34172503
28. Notarangelo G, Margelli M, Giovannico G, Bruno F, Milella C, Feller D, et al. Diagnostic utility of red flags for detecting spinal malignancies in patients with low back pain: a scoping

review. J Clin Med [Internet]. 2025;14(20) Available from: http://www.ncbi.nlm.nih.gov/pubmed/41156041
29. Miller J, West J, Khawar H, Middleton R. Cauda equina syndrome. Br J Hosp Med (Lond) [Internet]. 2023;84(11):1–7. Available from: http://www.ncbi.nlm.nih.gov/pubmed/38186331
30. Kavadichanda CG, Geng J, Bulusu SN, Negi VS, Raghavan M. Spondyloarthritis and the human leukocyte antigen (HLA)-B*27 connection. Front Immunol [Internet]. 2021;12:601518. Available from: http://www.ncbi.nlm.nih.gov/pubmed/33763060
31. Khan A, Bilezikian J. Primary hyperparathyroidism: pathophysiology and impact on bone. CMAJ [Internet]. 2000;163(2):184–7. Available from: http://www.ncbi.nlm.nih.gov/pubmed/10934983
32. Khalid N, Aeddula NR. Antineutrophil cytoplasmic antibodies (ANCA) test [Internet]. In: StatPearls; 2026. Available from: http://www.ncbi.nlm.nih.gov/pubmed/27481040.
33. Karne SS, Bhalerao NS. Carpal tunnel syndrome in hypothyroidism. J Clin Diagn Res [Internet]. 2016;10(2):OC36–8. Available from: http://www.ncbi.nlm.nih.gov/pubmed/27042500

Shoulder Soft Tissue Disorders

4

Abstract

Shoulder soft tissue disorders are common causes of shoulder pain, often presenting with overlapping symptoms of *rotator cuff tendinopathy*, *subacromial-subdeltoid bursitis, long head biceps tendinitis* and *adhesive capsulitis (frozen shoulder)*. This chapter uses a case-based approach to guide clinicians through shoulder anatomy, biomechanics, clinical presentation, examination, imaging, management and prognosis. Key anatomic concepts such as the rotator cuff muscles (supraspinatus, infraspinatus, teres minor and subscapularis) and the subacromial space are highlighted. We describe typical clinical features (e.g. painful arc of abduction, night pain, weakness and stiffness) and differentiate these soft tissue conditions from glenohumeral arthritis, cervical radiculopathy and systemic diseases like rheumatoid arthritis or polymyalgia rheumatica. Physical examination techniques (inspection, palpation, active/passive range of motion, strength testing and special tests such as Neer, Hawkins-Kennedy and Speed's) are detailed with evidence-based interpretation.

The role of imaging (X-ray, ultrasound, MRI) is explained, emphasising when each modality is indicated to confirm diagnosis or rule out other pathology. Management strategies are outlined: most cases respond to *conservative therapy* including activity modification, structured physiotherapy and analgesia, sometimes supplemented by targeted *injection therapy* (e.g. subacromial steroid or biceps sheath injection) if symptoms persist (Varacallo et al. Rotator cuff tendonitis [Internet]. In: StatPearls. Available from: http://www.ncbi.nlm.nih.gov/pubmed/29332181, 2026). Indications for surgical referral (e.g. refractory pain or weakness after ≥4–6 months of therapy) are given. Prognosis is generally favourable with proper treatment, although recovery may be protracted, especially in adhesive capsulitis which often follows a self-limited course (Li et al. Adhesive capsulitis (frozen shoulder) [Internet]. In: StatPearls. Available from: http://www.ncbi.nlm.nih.gov/pubmed/30451406, 2026). Throughout, a clinical case illustrates decision-making. This chapter is intended for rheumatologists,

© The Author(s), under exclusive license to Springer Nature Switzerland AG 2026

R. Amarnani, *Soft Tissue and Musculoskeletal Medicine in Rheumatology*,
https://doi.org/10.1007/978-3-032-29441-8_4

primary care and sports medicine clinicians dealing with shoulder pain, providing practical, up-to-date and case-based guidance.

Case Vignette

A 52-year-old right-hand-dominant woman presents with *gradual onset* of left shoulder pain over 3 months. She works as an accountant and recently took up tennis. She reports an "aching" pain in the front and side of her shoulder, especially with *overhead activities* (e.g. reaching up to shelves or serving in tennis) and at night when sleeping on that side. She denies true injury but recalls a minor fall on an outstretched arm 6 months ago. Over time, she finds it difficult to lift her arm above shoulder height, and her shoulder feels "stuck". There is no neck pain or numbness. She has tried ibuprofen and heat with modest relief. On examination, her posture is slightly guarded on the left, with mild muscle atrophy around the shoulder. Tenderness is present over the bicipital groove anteriorly and over the lateral aspect of the acromion. Active range of motion shows left shoulder abduction limited to 100° with pain (the classic *painful arc* between 60° and 120°) and passive range largely preserved. Passive forward flexion of the internally rotated arm reproduces pain, consistent with a positive Neer impingement sign. Hawkins-Kennedy testing, with the shoulder and elbow flexed to 90° followed by passive internal rotation, also reproduces pain. Strength testing shows slight weakness of supraspinatus and infraspinatus compared to the right. Spurling's test for cervical radiculopathy is negative. Preliminary diagnosis includes *subacromial impingement syndrome* (rotator cuff tendinopathy and bursitis) with possible biceps tendinitis. Adhesive capsulitis is considered due to her progressive stiffness. We will revisit this patient as we discuss examination, imaging and management.

Relevant Anatomy and Biomechanics

The shoulder complex comprises the glenohumeral joint, scapulothoracic articulation, acromioclavicular (AC) joint and sternoclavicular joint, working together to achieve a wide range of motion. The *glenohumeral joint* is a ball-and-socket joint with a large humeral head and small glenoid, granting high mobility but relying on soft tissues for stability [1]. Static stabilisers include the joint capsule, labrum and ligaments, while dynamic stabilisers are the rotator cuff muscles and long head of the biceps. The *rotator cuff* consists of four muscles (mnemonic "SITS"): *supraspinatus, infraspinatus, teres minor* and *subscapularis* [1]. These muscles arise from the scapula and insert around the proximal humerus, blending with the joint capsule to form a cuff that surrounds the joint. Their main biomechanical role is to compress the humeral head into the glenoid during motion, providing a stable fulcrum for shoulder movement [1]. In particular, supraspinatus initiates abduction (0–15°) and contributes to overhead stability, while infraspinatus and teres minor provide external rotation, and subscapularis provides internal rotation. Loss of rotator cuff function can lead to superior migration of the humeral head and impingement under the acromion.

The *subacromial-subdeltoid bursa* is a synovial-lined fluid sac beneath the acromion and deltoid, overlying the supraspinatus tendon and superior shoulder capsule [2]. It provides lubrication between the rotator cuff and acromion. The subacromial space can be approximately 1–1.5 cm in height [2], and any inflammation or narrowing (from tendon thickening, bursal inflammation, acromial morphology, acromioclavicular osteophytes or altered scapular mechanics) can cause impingement of the cuff and bursa. The *long head of the biceps tendon* originates from the superior glenoid labrum and supraglenoid tubercle, passes intraarticularly through the joint (in the rotator interval between subscapularis and supraspinatus) and exits via the bicipital groove of the humerus [3]. This tendon contributes to glenohumeral stability and is susceptible to overuse and impingement under the coracoacromial arch [3].

The *glenohumeral joint capsule* is loose and reinforced by the rotator cuff tendons. It is attached to the anatomic neck of the humerus and blends with the labrum. Key capsular ligaments (superior, middle and inferior glenohumeral ligaments and the coracohumeral ligament) limit extreme motion. Normal shoulder biomechanics require coordinated scapulothoracic motion (scapulohumeral rhythm), where the scapula rotates upward and posteriorly as the arm abducts, to maintain a stable subacromial clearance and optimise muscle length tension Fig. 4.1.

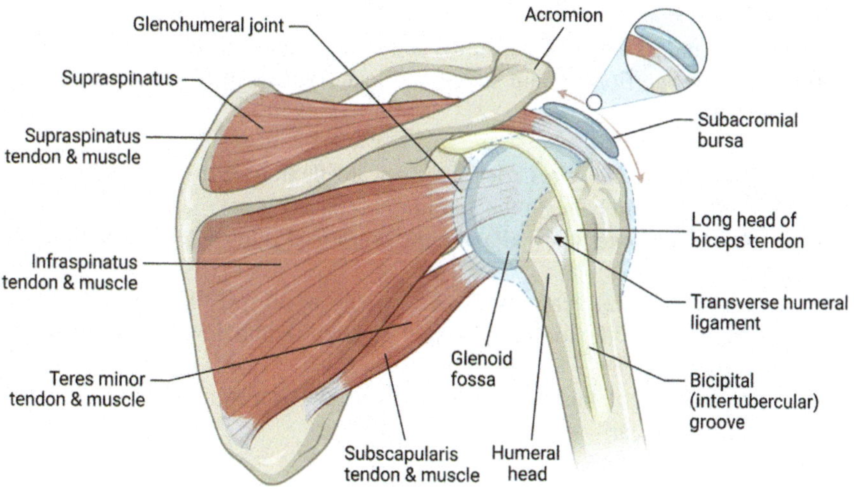

Fig. 4.1 Shoulder anatomy highlighting the glenohumeral joint, rotator cuff muscles, subacromial bursa and long head of biceps tendon

Clinical Presentation and Key Soft Tissue Pathologies

Rotator Cuff Tendinopathy (Supraspinatus/Infraspinatus)

Pathology
Rotator cuff tendinopathy refers to inflammation (tendinitis) or degeneration (tendinosis) of the rotator cuff tendons, most commonly the supraspinatus and sometimes infraspinatus [4]. It often occurs in association with subacromial impingement, where the tendon is repetitively pinched between the humeral head and acromial arch. Risk factors include overhead activities (e.g. throwing, swimming) and age-related undervascularised tendon regions (especially the supraspinatus footprint) [4]. Chronic impingement can lead to partial- or full-thickness tears over time.

Presentation
Patients typically report an *insidious onset* of shoulder pain exacerbated by overhead movements and lifting. Pain often localises to the lateral or posterior shoulder and may radiate down the arm but rarely below the elbow. A *painful arc* of abduction (usually between 60° and 120°) is characteristic [5]. Night pain (difficulty sleeping on the affected side) is common. Weakness with abduction and external rotation may develop as the condition progresses. Rotator cuff tendinopathy may follow acute trauma (a fall or lifting injury) or chronic overuse [6]. Middle-aged patients (40–60 years) and those with poor posture or scapular dyskinesis are often affected.

Examination Inspection may reveal localised swelling or muscle atrophy (especially of the supraspinatus or infraspinatus). Palpation often elicits point tenderness over the greater tuberosity (attachment of the supraspinatus) or along the anterior shoulder. Active range of motion (ROM) is limited by pain, whereas passive ROM is usually full (unless adhesive capsulitis is present). Notably, weakness with active motion out of proportion to pain suggests a tear. Typical special tests include the following [7]:

- *Neer impingement test:* Passive forward flexion of the internally rotated arm reproduces pain beneath the acromion.
- *Hawkins-Kennedy test:* Passive flexion to 90° with internal rotation elicits pain.
- *Jobe (empty can) test:* Weakness or pain when resisting downward pressure at 90° forward flexion in the scapular plane (thumb down) indicates supraspinatus involvement.
- *Drop arm test:* Inability to slowly lower the arm from 90° abduction suggests significant tear.

These tests are sensitive but not perfectly specific. Importantly, findings overlap with bursitis and impingement; in practice, a cluster of positive impingement signs

(Neer, Hawkins, painful arc) raises suspicion of rotator cuff pathology or subacromial bursitis.

Subacromial-Subdeltoid Bursitis

Pathology

The subacromial-subdeltoid bursa is a synovial cavity that can become inflamed (bursitis) from repetitive friction, impingement or direct trauma (Fig. 4.2). Common causes include chronic shoulder impingement, repetitive overhead activity (e.g. painting, weightlifting), direct falls, crystal deposition or rheumatoid arthritis [2]. Inflammation leads to bursal thickening and excess fluid, causing pain with shoulder movement. Because the bursa is contiguous with the coracoacromial arch structures, chronic bursitis often coexists with rotator cuff tendinopathy.

Presentation [2]

Bursitis presents very similarly to rotator cuff tendinopathy with lateral shoulder pain aggravated by overhead use. Patients often note tenderness directly under the acromion or over the deltoid. Pain is typically worse when raising the arm above the head and may also disturb sleep. Unlike adhesive capsulitis, passive motion is preserved (though painful), and weakness is usually mild. Systemic signs (e.g. warmth or redness) are absent unless infection or crystal disease is involved.

Examination Findings overlap greatly with rotator cuff disease. Palpation may reveal a broader tenderness over the anterolateral shoulder. The painful arc is again often present. Special tests for impingement (Neer, Hawkins) are usually positive.

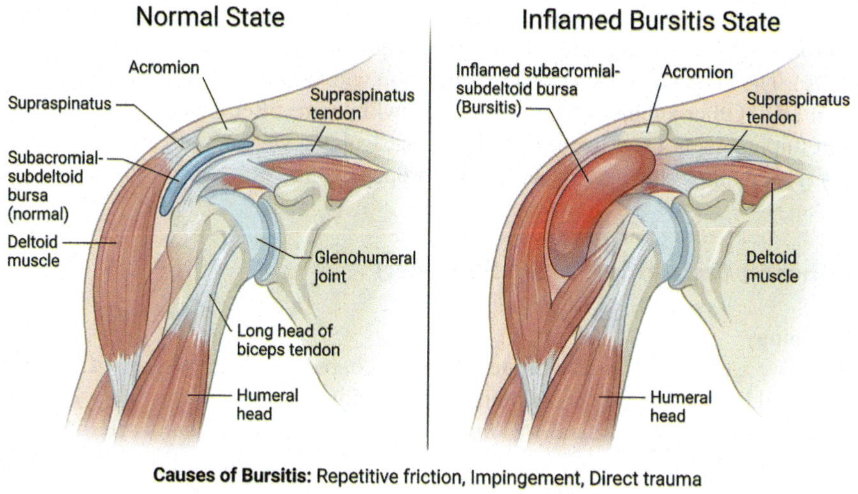

Fig. 4.2 Anatomy of shoulder subacromial bursitis and common causes

Because clinical distinction is difficult, bursitis is often diagnosed by excluding rotator cuff tears (via imaging) or by the response to a subacromial injection (symptomatic relief suggests a bursal or cuff cause).

Long Head Biceps Tendinitis

Pathology
Long head biceps tendinitis (and tendinosis) involves inflammation or degeneration of the biceps tendon, often within the bicipital groove [8]. It may be *primary* (isolated tendon pathology, ~5% of cases) or *secondary* to other shoulder problems (rotator cuff tears, SLAP lesions, scapular instability). Primary biceps impingement occurs when the tendon is pinched under the coracoacromial arch, often due to acromial spurs or thickened coracoacromial ligament. Overhead athletes and laborers are at risk, as are older patients with degenerative changes.

Presentation
Patients complain of a *deep, anterior shoulder ache* that can be difficult to localise. The pain often refers down the anterior arm and can mimic rotator cuff or cervical pain. Pain is often activity-related (lifting, pulling, throwing) and worsens at night, especially when lying on the affected arm. A classic sign is tenderness at the bicipital groove, exacerbated when the arm is in slight internal rotation (bringing the tendon forward in the groove). There may be a "snap" or catching sensation if the tendon subluxes or has an associated tear. Notably, isolated biceps tendinitis is often accompanied by rotator cuff pathology; only about 5% of biceps tendinitis occurs alone [9].

Examination The hallmark is *bicipital groove tenderness*. Speed's test involves resisted shoulder forward flexion with the elbow extended and forearm supinated, reproducing pain in the bicipital groove (though this has moderate sensitivity/specificity). The Yergason's test (resisted supination with elbow flexed) may also provoke pain [10]. Other shoulder exams (Neer, Hawkins) are often positive, since rotator cuff impingement usually coexists. However, isolated weakness in elbow flexion is not typical unless the tendon is ruptured (Popeye sign).

Adhesive Capsulitis (Frozen Shoulder)

Pathology
Adhesive capsulitis is a self-limited disorder characterised by global stiffening of the shoulder capsule due to inflammation and fibrosis. It occurs in about 2–5% of the population [11], classically in *middle-aged* individuals (mean onset ~55 years) and more often in women [12]. There are two types: primary (idiopathic, likely autoimmune or metabolic predisposition) and secondary (following trauma, surgery or immobilisation) [11]. Risk factors include *diabetes, thyroid disease, prolonged*

immobilisation and Parkinson's disease [13]. Frozen shoulder evolves in three phases: painful "freezing" phase (gradual onset of pain and stiffness, lasting ~3–9 months), adhesive "frozen" phase (extensive stiffness, ~4–12 months) and thawing phase (slow recovery of motion) (Fig. 4.3).

Presentation

Patients report progressive *diffuse shoulder pain and stiffness*, often bilateral, though one side dominates. Unlike rotator cuff problems, the pain in adhesive capsulitis is usually more constant (often worse at night) and is accompanied by a *marked loss of both active and passive ROM* in all planes, especially external rotation [12]. On exam, the hallmark is severely limited passive movement; if the arm cannot be passively rotated to near neutral, frozen shoulder is likely. The onset is insidious, without clear injury. Frozen shoulder is distinguished from glenohumeral osteoarthritis by the clinical capsular pattern, particularly marked loss of passive external rotation, and by preserved joint space on radiographs. In diabetics, onset can be bilateral and more refractory.

Examination Inspection may show a protective posture and muscle guarding. Active ROM is severely limited in flexion, abduction and rotation. Importantly, *passive external rotation is markedly reduced* [14]. This differentiates adhesive capsulitis from impingement (where passive ROM is normal) and glenohumeral OA (where motion is painful but often similarly limited). No specific special test "provokes" frozen shoulder; rather, a thorough ROM exam establishes the diagnosis by exclusion. A cervical screen, including Spurling's test where radicular symptoms are suspected, helps exclude cervical causes.

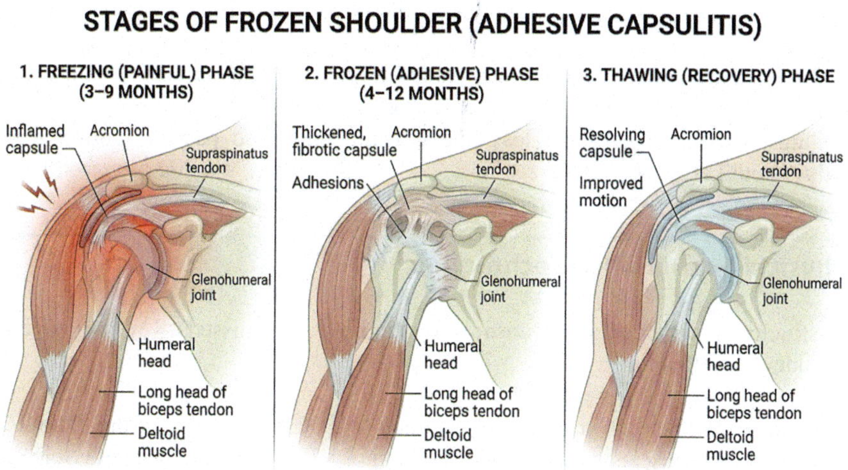

Fig. 4.3 Natural progression of adhesive capsulitis (frozen shoulder)

Differential Diagnosis of Shoulder Pain [15]

When evaluating shoulder pain, one must consider other causes beyond soft tissue disorders. Important differentials include the following:

- *Glenohumeral osteoarthritis:* Degenerative arthritis causes deep, aching pain, stiffness that worsens with use and crepitus. It often affects older patients. Exam shows limited passive motion but typically in a capsular pattern with internal rotation especially limited. X-ray shows joint space narrowing, osteophytes and subchondral sclerosis.
- *Cervical radiculopathy:* C5–C6 radiculopathy can mimic shoulder pain. Patients may have neck pain, arm dysesthesias in a dermatomal pattern and neurological signs. A Spurling manoeuvre (neck extension and rotation) that reproduces arm pain suggests a cervical source. Exam should include neck ROM, reflexes and upper limb neuro exam.
- *Acromioclavicular (AC) joint pathology:* AC joint arthritis or separation causes localised pain at the top of the shoulder, often provoked by cross-body adduction or palpation of the AC joint.
- *Labral tears (SLAP lesion):* Superior labrum tears (common in overhead athletes) can cause deep "clicking" pain, often with certain arm positions. Specific tests (O'Brien's, Speed's) may suggest labrum involvement.
- *Systemic inflammatory disease:* Conditions like rheumatoid arthritis or polymyalgia rheumatica (PMR) often involve the shoulder. RA causes joint synovitis with morning stiffness and multiple joint involvement. PMR classically presents in older adults with bilateral shoulder stiffness and elevated inflammatory markers. A careful history of systemic symptoms (fatigue, multiple joints) and lab tests (RF, ESR/CRP, ANA) help distinguish these.
- *Other shoulder pathology:* Frozen shoulder can mimic rotator cuff tear, but adhesive capsulitis has the described ROM pattern. Biceps tendon rupture (the Popeye deformity) causes acute bruising and relief of pain once ruptured.

Understanding these differentials guides appropriate tests (e.g. X-ray for arthritis) and avoids misdiagnosis. In our case, the lack of neck symptoms and unilateral findings made radiculopathy less likely, while preserved passive motion made arthritis unlikely.

Physical Examination Techniques

A structured shoulder exam ensures no findings are missed. Key components include the following:

- *Inspection:* Observe posture and symmetry. Look for atrophy of the deltoid or rotator cuff muscles, scapular winging, joint swelling or skin changes. Note any scars (previous surgery) or deformity (biceps rupture bulge, AC joint prominence).

- *Palpation:* Systematically palpate the shoulder girdle: the sternoclavicular joint, clavicle, AC joint, coracoid, greater and lesser tuberosities, bicipital groove, deltoid insertion and scapular spine. Tenderness over the *bicipital groove* suggests biceps tendinitis; tenderness at the *anterolateral acromion* suggests subacromial pathology. Crepitus or pain at the AC joint points to AC arthrosis.
- *Range of motion (ROM):* Assess *active and passive* ROM in flexion, abduction, internal and external rotation and extension. In rotator cuff impingement or bursitis, passive ROM is usually preserved though painful, whereas in adhesive capsulitis, both active and passive ROM (especially ER and abduction) are severely limited. The *painful arc* of 60–120° abduction is a hallmark of subacromial impingement. Document any pain or crepitus during motion.
- *Strength testing:* Test key muscles and nerve root levels (C5–T1). Key rotator cuff tests include the following:
  - *Supraspinatus (C5):* Jobe's (empty can) test and pain or weakness in resisted abduction at 90° can indicate supraspinatus injury.
  - *Infraspinatus/teres minor (C5–C6):* Resisted external rotation test and external rotation lag sign (arm at side, elbow flexed 90°, hold at external rotation and release; if it drifts inward, suspect tear).

    Subscapularis (C5–C6): Lift-off and belly-press tests for internal rotation weakness.
- *Special Tests for Impingement*
  - *Neer impingement test:* With scapula stabilised, passively flex the internally rotated arm fully. Pain indicates impingement of the rotator cuff under the acromion.
  - *Hawkins-Kennedy test:* Flex the shoulder and elbow to 90°, and then internally rotate. Pain suggests supraspinatus impingement.

    Painful arc: Have patient actively abduct the arm; pain between 60° and 120° supports subacromial impingement.
- *Special Tests for the Proximal Long Head of Biceps Tendon*
  - *Speed's test:* With elbow extended and forearm supinated, resist forward flexion of the shoulder. Pain in the bicipital groove indicates biceps tendon pathology (Speed's test).

    Yergason's test: With elbow flexed at 90° and palm down, resist supination. Pain at the groove is positive for biceps involvement.
- *Other tests:* Examine the AC joint by cross-arm adduction (Scarf testing); test scapular motion by having the patient push against a wall (winging suggests serratus anterior/paralysis). Importantly, do a *cervical spine exam:* check neck ROM, Spurling's test (head extension/rotation with downward pressure) and shoulder reflexes to screen for cervical radiculopathy.

This examination will yield a cluster of findings. For example, our patient had painful arc and positive Neer/Hawkins (suggesting impingement) with bicipital groove tenderness but no gross ROM restriction. This pattern fits subacromial pathology rather than adhesive capsulitis.

Role of Imaging

Imaging is used to confirm the suspected diagnosis, identify structural lesions or exclude other pathology. The choice depends on the clinical scenario:

- *X-ray:* Could be considered first line for chronic shoulder pain. A true *Grashey view* (true AP with scapula profile) is recommended to evaluate the glenohumeral joint [16]. X-rays can reveal osteoarthritis, humeral head sclerosis, subchondral cysts or glenoid changes. They also show acromion morphology (type III hook can predispose to impingement), AC joint osteoarthritis, calcific tendonitis (as calcifications) or other bony abnormalities. In suspected adhesive capsulitis, X-ray is typically normal or may show mild degenerative changes; its main role is to *rule out arthritis or fracture*.
- *Ultrasound:* A quick, dynamic and cost-effective tool. Shoulder ultrasound can visualise the rotator cuff tendons (detecting tears or thickening), bursal fluid and biceps tendon pathology. The sensitivity for large rotator cuff tears is high. Ultrasound can also guide injections.
- *Magnetic resonance imaging (MRI):* MRI is more sensitive for intraarticular structures. It can detect partial-thickness rotator cuff tears, labral tears, biceps anchor lesions (SLAP) and subtle glenohumeral joint pathology. MRI arthrography can also be especially useful for labral lesions. For suspected adhesive capsulitis, MRI may show *thickening of the coracohumeral ligament and joint capsule,* but it is not needed for diagnosis; it is mainly used to exclude alternative diagnoses.
- *Other:* For refractory cases, advanced imaging like MRI or CT arthrogram can be used. Routine lab testing (e.g. ESR/CRP, rheumatoid factor) is not indicated for routine tendonitis but may be ordered if a systemic inflammatory cause is suspected or to confirm PMR.

In our patient, an initial shoulder X-ray was normal (no arthritis). We arranged an ultrasound, which confirmed mild supraspinatus tendinosis without full-thickness tear and some bursal fluid. Cervical spine X-rays and exam remained unremarkable, supporting a shoulder source.

Management Strategies

Management of shoulder soft tissue disorders is tailored to the specific diagnosis, symptom severity and patient goals. In all cases, *conservative treatment* is the first line unless there is an urgent indication such as acute traumatic full-thickness cuff tear with pseudoparesis/pseudoparalysis, dislocation, fracture or infection. Key strategies include the following:

- *Activity modification:* Advise patients to avoid or temporarily reduce aggravating activities. For rotator cuff and biceps injuries, rest from overhead work or sports is important. Splinting or slinging is generally *not* recommended long term (risk of stiffness), except minimal support if needed for comfort.

- *Physiotherapy:* A supervised physiotherapy programme is the cornerstone of nonoperative treatment for most shoulder soft tissue conditions. The programme is individualised but typically includes the following:
  - *Range-of-motion exercises:* Especially in early stages of adhesive capsulitis to prevent worsening stiffness (pendulum exercises, wand stretching).
  - *Strengthening and stabilisation:* Focus on rotator cuff and periscapular muscles. Scapular stabilisation exercises (e.g. scapular retraction, low rows) and cuff strengthening (e.g. resisted external/internal rotation with bands) help restore biomechanics.
  - *Stretching:* For tight pectorals or posterior capsule (e.g. sleeper stretch) as needed.
  - *Modalities:* Heat, ice, ultrasound or electrical stimulation may be used adjunctively, though evidence is limited.

    Progression: Therapy is progressed slowly, emphasising technique and gradual load increase. Even partial-thickness tears or tendinopathy often respond well to rehabilitation alone [6].
- *Medications:*
  - *Analgesics/NSAIDs:* For symptomatic pain control. NSAIDs can reduce inflammation and pain short term, used alongside physiotherapy.

    Topical agents such as anti-inflammatory gels may help for superficial pain.
- *Injection therapy:* Corticosteroid injections can provide rapid pain relief, often allowing better participation in physiotherapy. Common injection sites include the following:
  - *Subacromial (subdeltoid) bursa injection:* A local steroid (e.g. depo-medrone 20–40 mg) with anaesthetic into the subacromial space can relieve impingement and bursitis pain. Multiple studies show short-term benefits, though long-term efficacy varies [17]. Ultrasound guidance improves accuracy.
  - *Glenohumeral joint injection:* Rarely indicated for isolated extra-articular soft tissue pain, but intra-articular corticosteroid injection or hydrodilatation may be used in adhesive capsulitis to reduce pain and improve capsular distension.
- *Further Interventions.*
  - *Hydrodilatation:* For adhesive capsulitis, some clinicians perform arthrographic capsular distension (injecting fluid/corticosteroid to stretch the capsule under imaging) in refractory cases [18].
  - *Surgery:* Referral to orthopaedics is indicated if *nonoperative management fails* (persistent pain/weakness after 3–6+ months) or if there is a large rotator cuff tear. For rotator cuff tears, surgical repair is considered for full-thickness tears in younger or active patients or symptomatic partial tears not responding to rehab [19]. Biceps tenodesis (reanchoring the tendon to the humerus) may be done if the biceps tendon is irreversibly torn or refractory to therapy, particularly in younger, active patients.

Adhesive capsulitis release: Arthroscopic capsular release (cutting tight capsule) is rarely needed but may be considered if severe stiffness persists despite aggressive physiotherapy.

In our patient's case, we advised avoidance of overhead work and started a structured physiotherapy programme focusing on rotator cuff and scapular exercises. After 6 weeks with partial improvement, we performed an ultrasound guided subacromial corticosteroid injection, which gave significant pain relief and improved range. By 3 months, her pain was minimal and ROM nearly normal.

Prognosis and Return to Function

With appropriate care, most patients with soft tissue shoulder disorders recover well, though timelines vary:

- *Rotator cuff/bursitis* [6]*:* Most cases improve substantially with 3–6 months of conservative therapy. Partial-thickness tears often improve with rehabilitation; even many full-thickness tears may become asymptomatic without surgery. In the literature, a "moderate" strength recommendation supports initial NSAIDs and exercise for rotator cuff syndromes [20]. Return to activity usually occurs gradually over weeks; light activities can resume in 2–4 weeks once pain improves, with full return (e.g. to sports) by 3–4 months if recovery is smooth. Chronic symptoms beyond 6 months warrant reevaluation.
- *Biceps tendinitis:* Similarly, response to rest, NSAIDs and physiotherapy is usually good over 2–3 months. If pain is relieved, full activity can resume. Tenodesis is a reliable solution if tendon rupture or refractory pain persists, with high success in young athletes [21].
- *Adhesive capsulitis:* This condition is *self-limiting* but slow. Many patients improve over 1–3 years. With diligent physiotherapy, patients may regain ~90% of motion by 1–2 years [11]. Early intervention reduces disability time. Diabetic patients may have a worse prognosis (longer course). Residual stiffness may persist mildly, but most return to baseline function.
- *Overall:* The key to a good outcome is setting expectations: full recovery is possible but may take months, especially if stiffness is involved. Patients should be reassured that physio*therapy and gradual loading* are effective and that surgery is rarely the first step. In chronic or refractory cases, multidisciplinary care (physiotherapy, sport and exercise medicine, orthopaedics) ensures optimal recovery.

In our case, the patient's prognosis was favourable. At 12 weeks from presentation, she regained full motion and returned to tennis at a reduced level. She continued home exercises for maintenance. We emphasised education about shoulder mechanics and the importance of posture and scapular control to prevent recurrence.

Integration of Case

Our initial vignette illustrates a typical overlap of subacromial impingement and mild biceps involvement in a middle-aged patient. Key decision points for such a patient include performing a thorough exam (as above) to identify impingement signs and exclude neck or systemic causes, obtaining baseline imaging (X-ray/ultrasound) to confirm soft tissue pathology and exclude arthritis and initiating conservative therapy. We combined rest from aggravating activities with a tailored physiotherapy programme (rotator cuff and scapular exercises) and used a targeted subacromial steroid injection when progress plateaued. Monitoring response over 6–12 weeks determined our next steps. Because our patient improved, surgical referral was not needed. This case will be revisited in the summary to highlight "real-world" application of the principles above.

Key Learning Points

- *Shoulder anatomy:* Stability is mainly due to soft tissues (rotator cuff, labrum, capsule). The rotator cuff ("SITS") and long head biceps tendon are key dynamic stabilisers. The subacromial bursa cushions these structures (see Fig. 4.1).
- *Differential diagnosis:* Always exclude cervical radiculopathy (perform Spurling's test) and glenohumeral arthritis (evaluate with X-ray) when assessing shoulder pain. Consider inflammatory arthritis in patients with systemic symptoms.
- *Clinical features:* Rotator cuff tendinopathy/bursitis presents with lateral shoulder pain, painful arc (60–120°) and positive impingement tests (Neer, Hawkins). Biceps tendinitis causes anterior pain and bicipital groove tenderness. Adhesive capsulitis features global stiffness with *restricted passive motion* (especially external rotation).
- *Examination:* Use a systematic approach—inspect, palpate, measure active/passive ROM, test strength and apply special tests. Note that weakness with intact passive ROM suggests a tendon tear, whereas limited passive ROM suggests capsule stiffness.
- *Imaging:* Start with X-ray to rule out bony lesions. Ultrasound is effective for rotator cuff and biceps pathology. MRI is reserved for complex cases or preoperative planning. Imaging is more to *rule out* other pathology than to diagnose simple tendonitis.
- *Management:* First line is *conservative*—patient education, rest/modification, physiotherapy and NSAIDs. Physiotherapy (exercise-based, strengthening rotator cuff and scapular stabilisers) is the mainstay. Consider corticosteroid injection if pain limits rehabilitation. Surgery is for refractory cases or significant tears.
- *Prognosis:* Most patients respond well; adhesive capsulitis, while self-limiting, can last up to 1–3 years but responds to therapy. Emphasise adherence to exercise and realistic timelines. Follow up to adjust treatment if progress is unsatisfactory.

References

1. Maruvada S, Madrazo-Ibarra A, Varacallo MA. Anatomy, rotator cuff [Internet]. In: StatPearls; 2026. Available from: http://www.ncbi.nlm.nih.gov/pubmed/28204962.
2. Faruqi T, Rizvi TJ. Subacromial bursitis [Internet]. In: StatPearls; 2026. Available from: http://www.ncbi.nlm.nih.gov/pubmed/22802986.
3. Diplock B, Hing W, Marks D. The long head of biceps at the shoulder: a scoping review. BMC Musculoskelet Disord [Internet]. 2023;24(1):232. Available from: http://www.ncbi.nlm.nih.gov/pubmed/36978047
4. Desmeules F, Roy J-S, Lafrance S, Charron M, Dubé M-O, Dupuis F, et al. Rotator cuff tendinopathy diagnosis, nonsurgical medical care, and rehabilitation: a clinical practice guideline. J Orthop Sports Phys Ther [Internet]. 2025;55(4):235–74. Available from: http://www.ncbi.nlm.nih.gov/pubmed/40165544
5. Creech JA, Busse A, Li D, Pinkerman S, Silver S. Shoulder impingement syndrome [Internet]. In: StatPearls; 2026. Available from: http://www.ncbi.nlm.nih.gov/pubmed/31141546.
6. Varacallo MA, El Bitar Y, Mair SD. Rotator cuff tendonitis [Internet]. In: StatPearls; 2026. Available from: http://www.ncbi.nlm.nih.gov/pubmed/29332181.
7. Tennent TD, Beach WR, Meyers JF. A review of the special tests associated with shoulder examination. Part I: the rotator cuff tests. Am J Sports Med [Internet]. 2003;31(1):154–60. Available from: http://www.ncbi.nlm.nih.gov/pubmed/12531773
8. Varacallo MA, Mair SD. Proximal biceps tendinitis and tendinopathy [Internet]. In: StatPearls; 2026. Available from: http://www.ncbi.nlm.nih.gov/pubmed/29337716.
9. Churgay CA. Diagnosis and treatment of biceps tendinitis and tendinosis. Am Fam Physician [Internet]. 2009;80(5):470–6. Available from: http://www.ncbi.nlm.nih.gov/pubmed/19725488
10. Holtby R, Razmjou H. Accuracy of the Speed's and Yergason's tests in detecting biceps pathology and SLAP lesions: comparison with arthroscopic findings. Arthroscopy [Internet]. 2004;20(3):231–6. Available from: http://www.ncbi.nlm.nih.gov/pubmed/15007311
11. Li D, St Angelo JM, Taqi M. Adhesive capsulitis (frozen shoulder) [Internet]. In: StatPearls; 2026. Available from: http://www.ncbi.nlm.nih.gov/pubmed/30451406.
12. Mullen JP, Hauer TM, Lau EN, Lin A. Adhesive capsulitis of the shoulder. Arthroscopy [Internet]. 2025;41(7):2176–8. Available from: http://www.ncbi.nlm.nih.gov/pubmed/40545326
13. Milgrom C, Novack V, Weil Y, Jaber S, Radeva-Petrova DR, Finestone A. Risk factors for idiopathic frozen shoulder. Isr Med Assoc J [Internet]. 2008;10(5):361–4. Available from: http://www.ncbi.nlm.nih.gov/pubmed/18605360
14. Vita F, Pederiva D, Tedeschi R, Spinnato P, Origlio F, Faldini C, et al. Adhesive capsulitis: the importance of early diagnosis and treatment. J Ultrasound [Internet]. 2024;27(3):579–87. Available from: http://www.ncbi.nlm.nih.gov/pubmed/38844748
15. Greenberg DL. Evaluation and treatment of shoulder pain. Med Clin North Am [Internet]. 2014;98(3):487–504. Available from: http://www.ncbi.nlm.nih.gov/pubmed/24758957
16. Koh KH, Han KY, Yoon YC, Lee SW, Yoo JC. True anteroposterior (Grashey) view as a screening radiograph for further imaging study in rotator cuff tear. J shoulder Elb Surg [Internet]. 2013;22(7):901–7. Available from: http://www.ncbi.nlm.nih.gov/pubmed/23312822
17. Yatish R, Ashok Kumar BK, Suvarna AA, Channappa TS, Jayaram M, Shivakumar HB. Effect of ultrasound-guided subacromial Bursa injections with various doses of corticosteroid in subacromial bursitis: a retrospective study. Cureus [Internet]. 2025;17(8):e89307. Available from: http://www.ncbi.nlm.nih.gov/pubmed/40766090
18. Poku D, Hassan R, Migliorini F, Maffulli N. Efficacy of hydrodilatation in frozen shoulder: a systematic review and meta-analysis. Br Med Bull [Internet]. 2023;147(1):121–47. Available from: http://www.ncbi.nlm.nih.gov/pubmed/37496207
19. Kaptan AY, Ulucaköy C, Özer M, Çetinkaya M, Ayanoğlu T, Ataoğlu MB, et al. Partial and full-thickness rotator cuff tears in patients younger than 45 years. Acta Orthop Traumatol Turc [Internet]. 2020;54(5):478–82. Available from: http://www.ncbi.nlm.nih.gov/pubmed/33155555

20. Schwitzguébel AJ-P. Rotator cuff disorders: practical recommendations for conservative management based on the literature. Medicina (Kaunas) [Internet]. 2026;62(2) Available from: http://www.ncbi.nlm.nih.gov/pubmed/41752672
21. Belk JW, Kraeutler MJ, Houck DA, Chrisman AN, Scillia AJ, McCarty EC. Biceps tenodesis versus tenotomy: a systematic review and meta-analysis of level I randomized controlled trials. J Shoulder Elb Surg [Internet]. 2021;30(5):951–60. Available from: http://www.ncbi.nlm.nih.gov/pubmed/33373685

5 Elbow Pain and Epicondylitis

Abstract

Elbow pain is a frequent complaint in sport and exercise medicine, rheumatology and primary care. It often arises from overuse disorders such as lateral epicondylitis ("tennis elbow") and medial epicondylitis ("golfer's elbow"), which are tendinopathies of the extensor and flexor muscle origins, respectively. Other conditions including olecranon bursitis and distal biceps tendinopathy also cause characteristic elbow pain syndromes. This chapter reviews relevant elbow anatomy and biomechanics and presents a clinical case to illustrate common presentation. Key physical examination manoeuvres (e.g. Cozen's test, Mill's test, resisted wrist flexion, hook test) and appropriate imaging modalities (X-ray, ultrasound, MRI) are described. Conservative management is emphasised: activity modification, bracing, anti-inflammatory therapy and structured physiotherapy (notably eccentric strengthening) are first line. Injection therapies are reviewed; corticosteroids often yield short-term relief, whereas platelet-rich plasma (PRP) may offer longer-term benefit in chronic cases. Indications for surgical referral (e.g. persistent symptoms beyond 6–12 months or tendon rupture) are outlined. Prognosis is generally favourable; most patients recover with nonoperative care. Key learning points summarise practical takeaways for clinicians managing elbow soft tissue disorders.

Case Vignette

A 42-year-old right-handed carpenter presents with a 6-month history of gradually worsening pain over the lateral aspect of his right elbow. He reports that the pain began after an extended period of intense work using heavy hand tools. The pain is aggravated by gripping objects and by resisted wrist extension (e.g. using a power drill or lifting heavy materials). He also notes difficulty carrying a coffee mug or shaking hands without discomfort. On examination, there is focal tenderness just

© The Author(s), under exclusive license to Springer Nature Switzerland AG 2026

R. Amarnani, *Soft Tissue and Musculoskeletal Medicine in Rheumatology*,
https://doi.org/10.1007/978-3-032-29441-8_5

distal to the right lateral epicondyle, and pain is reproduced by resisted wrist extension. Grip strength on the affected side is modestly reduced. There is no swelling, erythema or neurovascular deficit. This scenario exemplifies the classic presentation of lateral epicondylitis, which affects an estimated 1–3% of adults annually and is common in labourers and athletes engaging in repetitive wrist-extension activities.

Relevant Anatomy and Biomechanics of the Elbow Joint

Anatomically, the elbow comprises three articulations: the humeroulnar and humeroradial joints (forming a hinge for flexion/extension) and the proximal radioulnar joint (allowing forearm pronation/supination) (Fig. 5.1) [1]. The distal humerus has medial and lateral epicondyles as attachment sites for forearm muscle tendons. The elbow's collateral ligaments (ulnar collateral ligament medially, radial collateral ligament laterally) and the osseous geometry (trochlea on ulna, capitellum on radius) provide stability. The radial nerve courses near the lateral epicondyle (on the anterior aspect of the joint), whereas the ulnar nerve lies in the cubital tunnel behind the medial epicondyle [1].

Biomechanically, repetitive forearm muscle use creates large stresses at these epicondylar origins. For example, repeated forceful wrist extension (as in weightlifting or racket sports) loads the extensor carpi radialis brevis tendon at the lateral epicondyle. Similarly, repeated wrist flexion or pronation (as in golf swings or swinging a hammer) stresses the flexor-pronator tendons at the medial epicondyle.

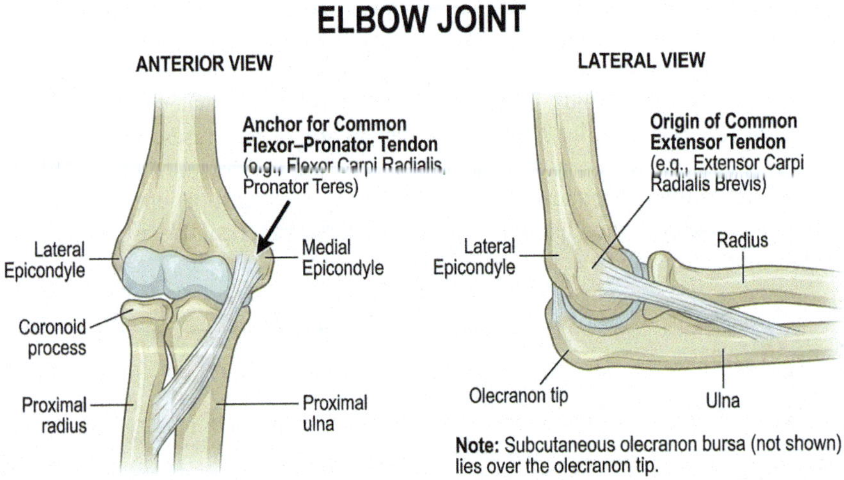

Fig. 5.1 Schematic views of the elbow joint (distal humerus, proximal radius/ulna and epicondyles) in anterior (left) and lateral (right) orientations. The lateral epicondyle serves as the origin of the common extensor tendon (e.g. extensor carpi radialis brevis) and the medial epicondyle anchors the common flexor-pronator tendon (including flexor carpi radialis and pronator teres). The subcutaneous olecranon bursa (not shown) lies over the olecranon tip

Overuse can lead to microtears and angiofibroblastic degeneration of the tendon (a tendinosis) rather than acute inflammation [2]. Understanding these attachments explains why lateral epicondylitis causes lateral elbow pain with resisted extension, while medial epicondylitis causes medial pain with resisted flexion.

Common Soft Tissue Conditions (Fig. 5.2)

Lateral Epicondylitis (Tennis Elbow)

Lateral epicondylitis is an overuse tendinopathy of the common extensor tendon at the lateral epicondyle. It affects roughly 1–3% of adults (typically aged 35–54) [3]. Activities involving repetitive wrist extension (e.g. tennis, painting, carpentry with power tools) are common causes. Histologically, the tendon shows chronic degeneration (angiofibroblastic changes) rather than acute inflammation. Clinically, patients have insidious lateral elbow pain that is aggravated by gripping and by resisted wrist extension [4]. Grip strength is often reduced. On exam, point tenderness is found at the lateral epicondyle. Special manoeuvres reproduce pain: Cozen's test (resisted wrist extension with elbow extended) and Mill's test (passive stretching of the wrist extensors) both elicit lateral elbow pain.

Medial Epicondylitis (Golfer's Elbow)

Medial epicondylitis involves chronic tendinosis of the flexor-pronator origin at the medial epicondyle. It is much less common than lateral epicondylitis. The condition

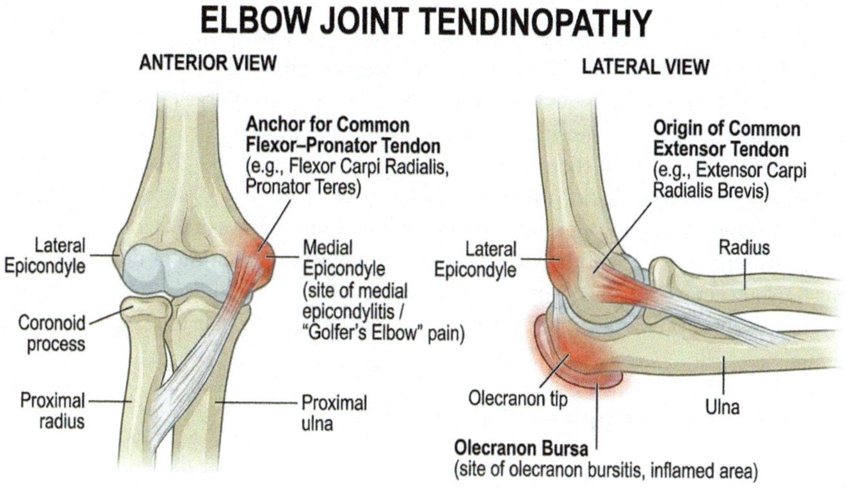

Fig. 5.2 Common sites of elbow tendinopathy and bursitis, including lateral epicondyle pain, medial epicondyle pain and the olecranon bursa

often arises from repetitive elbow valgus stress and forceful wrist flexion/pronation (e.g. golf swings, racket forehand strokes, hammering). Pathology shows degeneration of the common flexor tendon (especially flexor carpi radialis and pronator teres) at the medial epicondyle [5]. Patients report medial elbow pain which is reproduced by resisted wrist flexion and forearm pronation on exam. There is point tenderness just anterior to the medial epicondyle. Symptoms can radiate into the forearm. Paraesthesia in the ulnar distribution may occur, but true sensory loss is uncommon unless an ulnar neuropathy coexists.

Olecranon Bursitis

Olecranon bursitis is inflammation of the subcutaneous bursa overlying the olecranon. It often results from repetitive minor trauma or pressure (e.g. leaning on elbows), prolonged elbow flexion or occasionally infection. Patients present with posterior elbow swelling. In *aseptic bursitis*, the swelling is typically painless or only mildly tender without erythema. In *septic bursitis*, the patient has severe pain, redness, warmth over the olecranon and systemic symptoms (approximately 50% have fever) [6]. Diagnosis of septic vs aseptic is confirmed by aspirating bursal fluid (Gram stain and culture). Management of aseptic bursitis is conservative (padding, compression, NSAIDs (non-steroidal anti-inflammatory drugs), activity modification). A systematic review found nonoperative treatment (aspiration and bandaging) to be effective and safer than surgery [7]. Corticosteroid injection into the bursa is generally avoided because it carries a high risk of skin atrophy and infection [7]. Surgical bursectomy is reserved for chronic, refractory cases or uncontrolled infection.

Distal Biceps Tendinopathy

Distal biceps tendinopathy is a source of anterior elbow pain from chronic overload of the distal biceps tendon. Complete distal biceps ruptures are rare (~3% of tendon ruptures), but partial tears and tendinopathy are more common [8]. Patients typically complain of deep anterior elbow pain and weakness in forearm supination or elbow flexion. On exam there is tenderness in the antecubital fossa, and resisted supination (or elbow flexion) reproduces the pain. The "hook" test (palpating the biceps tendon in full supination) remains positive in tendinopathy, confirming tendon continuity. Ultrasound or MRI can confirm tendon thickening or detect a partial tear. Distal biceps tendinopathy is managed nonoperatively unless a full-thickness tear is present; complete ruptures usually require surgical repair to restore function.

Clinical Presentation and Differentiation [9]

Accurate diagnosis depends on localising pain to specific structures. Lateral epicondylitis produces lateral elbow pain exacerbated by gripping or resisted wrist extension. Medial epicondylitis yields medial elbow pain aggravated by wrist flexion/pronation. Olecranon bursitis causes a palpable posterior swelling; presence of erythema, warmth or fever suggests infection. Distal biceps tendinopathy causes deep anterior elbow pain with resisted supination or flexion. Differential diagnoses include nerve entrapments: radial tunnel syndrome can mimic lateral epicondylitis (pain often a few centimetres distal to the epicondyle and not clearly provoked by wrist extension), whereas cubital tunnel syndrome (ulnar neuropathy) can mimic medial epicondylitis (look for numbness in the ring/little fingers and Tinel's sign at the elbow). Inflammatory arthritis or gout can cause more diffuse elbow pain. In overhead athletes, valgus-extension overload (posterior impingement) in throwers should be considered. In practice, careful reproduction of symptoms with specific tests (and noting the exact location of pain) usually reveals the correct diagnosis.

Physical Examination Techniques

A focused elbow exam confirms the diagnosis. Begin with palpation: the lateral epicondyle and common extensor tendon origin are tender in tennis elbow, while the medial epicondyle area is tender in golfer's elbow. The key provocative tests are the following:

- *Cozen's test (tennis elbow)*: With the elbow extended and forearm pronated, the patient makes a fist and resists wrist extension. Pain at the lateral epicondyle is a positive sign. Cozen's test has very high sensitivity (about 91%) [10].
- *Mill's test (tennis elbow)*: The examiner passively pronates the forearm, flexes the wrist fully and then extends the elbow. This stretches the wrist extensor origin and elicits pain in lateral epicondylitis. Mill's test sensitivity is roughly 87% [11].
- *Maudsley's test*: The patient resists extension of the middle finger with the wrist flexed. Pain over the lateral epicondyle suggests tendon overload [11].
- *Golfer's elbow test*: The elbow is extended and forearm supinated; resisting wrist flexion/pronation reproduces medial elbow pain in medial epicondylitis [2].
- *Hook test (distal biceps)*: With the shoulder abducted and elbow at 90°, the examiner attempts to "hook" a finger under the biceps tendon at the antecubital fossa. Inability to hook (tendon not palpable) indicates a complete distal biceps tear [12].

Neurological examination is also important: check radial nerve function (wrist/ finger extension, Tinel's at radial tunnel) and ulnar nerve function (ring/ little finger sensation, elbow Tinel's) to rule out neuropathies. Assess range of motion and stability; for example, valgus stress testing may be relevant in throwers.

Imaging Modalities and Indications

Plain Radiography Obtain elbow X-rays (AP and lateral) if trauma is suspected or to rule out bony lesions or arthritis. X-rays can identify fractures, osteophytes, joint space changes or calcifications. In olecranon bursitis, an X-ray can detect an olecranon fracture or osteomyelitis.

Ultrasound This is a useful, quick and inexpensive modality for soft tissues. Ultrasound can dynamically assess tendon thickness, tears, neovascularity and fluid collections. It can confirm tendonitis, partial tears or bursitis in real time. For example, an ultrasound can show thickening of the common extensor origin in tennis elbow or bursal fluid collection in bursitis.

MRI MRI is preferred for chronic or complicated cases. It provides high-resolution images of soft tissues, showing the extent of tendinosis, partial or complete tears and muscle atrophy. MRI is indicated if symptoms persist despite 3–6 months of treatment, to assess for tendon tears, cartilage injury or other pathology. It is often obtained preoperatively to plan surgery. In summary, X-ray is the first line modality (to rule out fracture/arthritis), ultrasound is used for screening tendon pathology, and MRI is helpful when deeper or more comprehensive evaluation is needed.

Conservative Management

First-line treatment is usually conservative. *Activity modification* is important: avoid or adjust aggravating motions (e.g. reduce repetitive wrist extension or flexion). *Pain control* includes ice application, nonsteroidal antiinflammatory drugs (NSAIDs) or paracetamol. A *counterforce brace* (tennis elbow strap) applied just distal to the epicondyle may offload the tendon and improve grip strength. Short-term wrist immobilisation (in mild extension) can relieve acute symptoms.

Physiotherapy is the cornerstone of rehabilitation. A supervised programme emphasising *eccentric strengthening* of the involved muscle group has shown the greatest benefit in lateral epicondylitis [3]. For tennis elbow, eccentric wrist extension exercises with progressively increasing resistance are advised; for golfer's elbow, eccentric wrist flexion exercises are used. Stretching of the wrist extensors or flexors and forearm pronators/supinators is also important. Manual therapy (soft tissue mobilisation, cross-friction massage) may be adjunctive. Gradual return to full activity is guided by symptom tolerance. Address ergonomic factors (workplace setup or sports technique).

Other modalities have limited evidence, for example, shockwave therapy and steroid injections are not first line. In *olecranon bursitis*, conservative care (elbow padding, compression bandaging, avoiding pressure on the elbow, NSAIDs) usually suffices; bursal aspiration with compression dressing can help if painful. *Return to activity* is individualised: as pain allows, patients may resume sports or manual work with gradual progression. With diligent conservative care, many patients often improve over weeks to months.

Role of Corticosteroid and Platelet-Rich Plasma Injections

Corticosteroid injection around the painful tendon origin or into an inflamed bursa can provide rapid relief, but benefits are usually short-lived. Meta-analyses show that corticosteroids outperform other treatments at 1–2 months, but by 6–12 months, they no longer provide superior benefit [13]. Thus, steroids may be offered for rapid short-term relief, especially if symptoms are severe, but patients should be warned of potential recurrence. Steroid injections also risk tendon weakening or skin atrophy and should generally be limited where possible. For example, steroid injection into an olecranon bursa is associated with a high complication rate [7].

Platelet-rich plasma (PRP) injections have become popular for chronic epicondylitis. PRP is thought to promote healing by delivering growth factors. Recent trials and systematic reviews suggest that PRP yields better long-term pain relief and functional improvement than corticosteroids in epicondylitis [14]. In practice, PRP is usually reserved for chronic cases (symptoms >6–12 months) or after failure of more conservative measures. The procedure involves ultrasound-guided injection of autologous platelet concentrate into the degenerative tendon. Early evidence supports PRP as a reasonable option for refractory epicondylitis. Other injections (autologous whole blood, prolotherapy) have been studied but have weaker evidence [15].

Indications for Surgical Referral

Surgery is reserved for a small minority of patients. If symptoms persist despite 6–12 months of comprehensive nonoperative care, surgical intervention may be considered. In refractory lateral or medial epicondylitis, operative options include open or arthroscopic release of the diseased tendon origin, often with debridement of degenerative tissue. Only about 5–10% of epicondylitis patients eventually undergo surgery [4]. Complete distal biceps tendon ruptures (especially acute tears in young, active patients) are typically repaired surgically to restore elbow flexion and forearm supination strength. Chronic tears in older or low-demand patients may sometimes be managed nonoperatively. Olecranon bursitis rarely requires surgery; bursectomy is indicated only for chronic recalcitrant bursitis or uncontrolled infection after exhausting conservative measures.

Prognosis and Return to Activity Expectations

Prognosis is generally favourable. With appropriate management, most patients gradually improve. In one large study of tennis elbow, approximately 90% of patients reported significant relief at 1 year with nonoperative care [4]. Complete recovery may take many months, and patients should be counselled to adhere to therapy. Medial epicondylitis has a similar time course. Olecranon bursitis usually resolves completely with rest and treatment (antibiotics if septic). Distal biceps tendinopathy typically responds to therapy as well. If surgical repair of a biceps tear is performed, patients usually begin gentle active motion by 3–4 months and can expect to regain full strength by 6–9 months postoperatively.

Key Learning Points

- *Elbow tendinopathy*: The most common causes of chronic elbow pain are lateral and medial epicondylitis, affecting the extensor and flexor tendons respectively. Consider the activity pattern (repeated extension vs flexion) when localising pain.
- *Examination*: Provocative tests are key. Cozen's and Mill's tests reproduce pain in tennis elbow, while resisted wrist flexion/pronation elicits golfer's elbow pain. The Hook test checks distal biceps integrity. Positive findings should correspond to the patient's pain location.
- *Imaging*: Begin with X-rays to exclude fracture, arthritis or bony avulsion. Use ultrasound and MRI selectively: ultrasound is excellent for confirming tendon pathology or bursitis dynamically; MRI is most helpful in chronic or unclear cases.
- *Nonoperative treatment*: First-line management is conservative. Activity modification, NSAIDs/ice and counterforce bracing can relieve symptoms. A structured rehabilitation programme with progressive eccentric loading and stretching of the affected muscle group yields the best outcomes.
- *Injection therapies*: Corticosteroid injections may offer short-term pain relief but do not improve long-term outcome. PRP injection has shown better long-term improvement in chronic epicondylitis and may be considered if initial treatments fail. Other injections have less evidence.
- *Surgery*: Reserved for recalcitrant cases. Only about 5–10% of epicondylitis patients require surgery. Surgical release of the tendon origin is considered after 6–12 months of failed therapy. Complete distal biceps ruptures typically warrant surgical repair for full return of strength.
- *Prognosis*: Most patients improve with time. About 90% of tennis elbow patients improve by 1 year, although full recovery can take longer. Emphasise gradual return to activity and continued adherence to exercise therapy.

References

1. Alcid JG, Ahmad CS, Lee TQ. Elbow anatomy and structural biomechanics. Clin Sports Med. 2004;23(4):503–17, vii. Available from: http://www.ncbi.nlm.nih.gov/pubmed/15474218.
2. Reece CL, Li D, Susmarski AJ. Medial epicondylitis. StatPearls; 2026. Available from: https://www.ncbi.nlm.nih.gov/books/NBK557869/.

3. Landesa-Piñeiro L, Leirós-Rodríguez R. Physiotherapy treatment of lateral epicondylitis: a systematic review. J Back Musculoskelet Rehabil. 2022;35(3):463–77. Available from: http://www.ncbi.nlm.nih.gov/pubmed/34397403.
4. Zhang C, Jia Z, Li J, Wang X, Yang S. Impact of lifestyle and clinical factors on the prognosis of tennis elbow. Sci Rep. 2024;14(1):3063. Available from: http://www.ncbi.nlm.nih.gov/pubmed/38321129.
5. Li D, Hammad A, Kaiser K. Medial epicondylitis (Golfer's elbow). StatPearls; 2026. Available from: https://www.ncbi.nlm.nih.gov/books/NBK519000/.
6. Pangia J, Taqi M, Rizvi TJ. Olecranon bursitis. StatPearls; 2026. Available from: http://www.ncbi.nlm.nih.gov/pubmed/26577126.
7. Sayegh ET, Strauch RJ. Treatment of olecranon bursitis: a systematic review. Arch Orthop Trauma Surg. 2014;134(11):1517–36. Available from: http://www.ncbi.nlm.nih.gov/pubmed/25234151.
8. Kolaczko JG, Knapik DM, McMellen CJ, Mengers SR, Gillespie RJ, Voos JE. Complete isolated ruptures of the distal biceps Brachii during athletic activity: a systematic review. Cureus. 2022;14(8):e27899. Available from: http://www.ncbi.nlm.nih.gov/pubmed/35971400.
9. Tham J-L, Al-Ani Z. Elbow pain and clicking. Skeletal Radiol. 2022;51(11):2229–31. Available from: http://www.ncbi.nlm.nih.gov/pubmed/35376982.
10. Karanasios S, Korakakis V, Moutzouri M, Drakonaki E, Koci K, Pantazopoulou V, et al. Diagnostic accuracy of examination tests for lateral elbow tendinopathy (LET) – a systematic review. J Hand Ther. 2022;35(4):541–51. Available from: http://www.ncbi.nlm.nih.gov/pubmed/33814224.
11. Greene C, Droppelmann G, García N, Jorquera C, Verdugo A. A new test for the advanced diagnosis of lateral elbow tendinopathy with concomitant Intrasubstance tear: failure to resist extension effort (the free test). Orthop Res Rev. 2022;14:495–503. Available from: http://www.ncbi.nlm.nih.gov/pubmed/36606066.
12. O'Driscoll SW, Goncalves LBJ, Dietz P. The hook test for distal biceps tendon avulsion. Am J Sports Med. 2007;35(11):1865–9. Available from: http://www.ncbi.nlm.nih.gov/pubmed/17687121.
13. Johnson GW, Cadwallader K, Scheffel SB, Epperly TD. Treatment of lateral epicondylitis. Am Fam Physician. 2007;76(6):843–8. Available from: http://www.ncbi.nlm.nih.gov/pubmed/17910298.
14. Xu Y, Li T, Wang L, Yao L, Li J, Tang X. Platelet-rich plasma has better results for long-term functional improvement and pain relief for lateral epicondylitis: a systematic review and meta-analysis of randomized controlled trials. Am J Sports Med. 2024;52(10):2646–56. Available from: http://www.ncbi.nlm.nih.gov/pubmed/38357713.
15. Hohmann E, Tetsworth K, Glatt V. Corticosteroid injections for the treatment of lateral epicondylitis are superior to platelet-rich plasma at 1 month but platelet-rich plasma is more effective at 6 months: an updated systematic review and meta-analysis of level 1 and 2 studies. J Shoulder Elb Surg. 2023;32(9):1770–83. Available from: http://www.ncbi.nlm.nih.gov/pubmed/37247780.

6 Hand and Wrist: Tendinopathies and Entrapment Syndromes

Abstract

Hand and wrist pain from tendinopathies and nerve entrapment is common in rheumatologic practice. This chapter reviews the functional anatomy of tendons and nerves in the wrist and hand and describes common soft tissue disorders affecting this region. De Quervain's tenosynovitis (a stenosing disorder of the first dorsal extensor compartment), trigger finger (stenosing flexor tenosynovitis) and carpal tunnel syndrome are covered in detail, along with other nerve compression syndromes such as ulnar (Guyon canal) and radial (posterior interosseous) neuropathies. We discuss how to distinguish mechanical overuse syndromes from inflammatory arthropathies (e.g. rheumatoid arthritis, gout) by history and exam. Key special tests (Finkelstein's for De Quervain's, Phalen's and Tinel's for carpal tunnel, etc.) and diagnostic tools (ultrasound, nerve conduction studies, MRI) are reviewed. Management strategies are then outlined: conservative care including splinting, activity modification, NSAIDs and physiotherapy, injection therapies (corticosteroid, hydrodissection) often under ultrasound guidance and indications for surgical referral when symptoms are severe or refractory. Prognosis and long-term outcomes are summarised for each condition. Throughout, clinical pearls and illustrative figure (e.g. flexor pulley anatomy, transverse carpal ligament) are provided to reinforce anatomy and pathophysiology.

Clinical Vignette

A 32-year-old right-hand-dominant woman presents 6 months postpartum with insidious onset of pain at the radial side of her right wrist. She reports that picking up her 4-month-old baby repeatedly aggravates the pain, which is worse when she moves or grips with the thumb. She denies neck pain or systemic symptoms. On exam, there is tenderness at the right radial styloid, with mild swelling and pain radiating into the thumb. Active thumb extension and abduction reproduce her pain.

© The Author(s), under exclusive license to Springer Nature Switzerland AG 2026

R. Amarnani, *Soft Tissue and Musculoskeletal Medicine in Rheumatology*,
https://doi.org/10.1007/978-3-032-29441-8_6

There is no wrist instability or ulnar-sided symptoms. Finkelstein's test is positive (pain with forced ulnar deviation while the thumb is flexed across the palm). The rest of her musculoskeletal and neurologic exam is unremarkable. A provisional diagnosis of postpartum de Quervain's tenosynovitis is made, given the classic exam findings and history of repetitive thumb use with infant care. Initial management includes thumb spica splinting and a trial of oral NSAIDs and activity modification. After 4 weeks, she has only modest improvement and remains symptomatic with caring for her baby. An ultrasound-guided corticosteroid injection into the first dorsal compartment is then performed, which provides near-complete pain relief within 2 weeks.

Functional Anatomy of the Wrist and Hand [1]

The hand and wrist are a complex composite of bones, joints, tendons, muscles and nerves that permit fine motor function. The distal radius and ulna articulate with eight carpal bones arranged in two rows, forming the wrist joint. The carpal tunnel is a fibroosseous canal on the palmar (volar) side of the wrist: its floor and sides are formed by the carpal bones (especially the scaphoid and lunate) and its roof by the transverse carpal ligament (flexor retinaculum) (Fig. 6.1). The carpal tunnel contains the median nerve and nine flexor tendons (the four flexor digitorum profundus, four flexor digitorum superficialis and the flexor pollicis longus). Compression

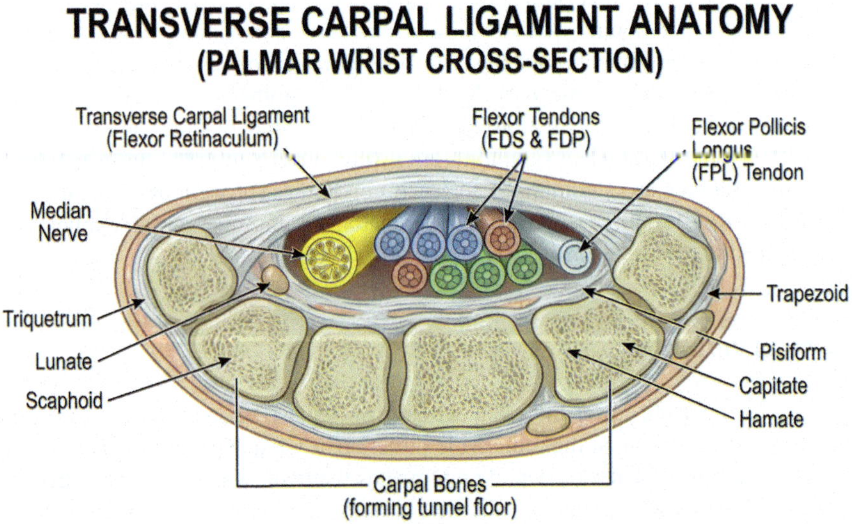

Fig. 6.1 Transverse carpal ligament anatomy (view of palmar wrist cross-section showing the carpal tunnel floor (carpal bones) and roof (flexor retinaculum) with median nerve and flexor tendons)

within this space (e.g. by tenosynovial swelling or ligament thickening) causes median neuropathy (carpal tunnel syndrome).

The flexor tendons of the fingers are held close to the bones by a series of annular and cruciform pulleys (fibrous bands) that form the digital flexor sheath. In each finger, there are five annular pulleys (A1 at the metacarpophalangeal joint down to A5 at the distal interphalangeal joint) and three cruciate pulleys [2]. For example, the A1 pulley is a transverse band over the base of the finger; its proximal edge arises from the volar plate of the metacarpophalangeal joint and it extends to the base of the proximal phalanx. The A2 and A4 pulleys lie along the proximal and middle phalanges and are the major load-bearing pulleys. The A3 pulley overlies the proximal interphalangeal joint (see Fig. 6.2: Flexor pulley system of the fingers). The thumb has a simplified system with only two pulleys (A1 and A2). These pulleys prevent bowstringing of the flexor tendons and maintain normal tendon tension during finger flexion. In trigger finger (stenosing tenosynovitis), the A1 pulley typically becomes thickened relative to the underlying flexor tendons, leading to catching and locking of the digit [3].

On the dorsal (back) side of the wrist, the six extensor compartments are numbered from radial to ulnar. The first dorsal compartment at the radial styloid contains the tendons of abductor pollicis longus (APL) and extensor pollicis brevis (EPB). De Quervain's tenosynovitis is inflammation of this first compartment (affecting the APL and EPB tendons) causing pain at the radial wrist [4]. The second through sixth compartments contain the other extensor tendons (extensor carpi radialis longus, brevis in compartment 2, etc.). Tenderness or crepitus over a given compartment suggests tenosynovitis of the tendons in that compartment.

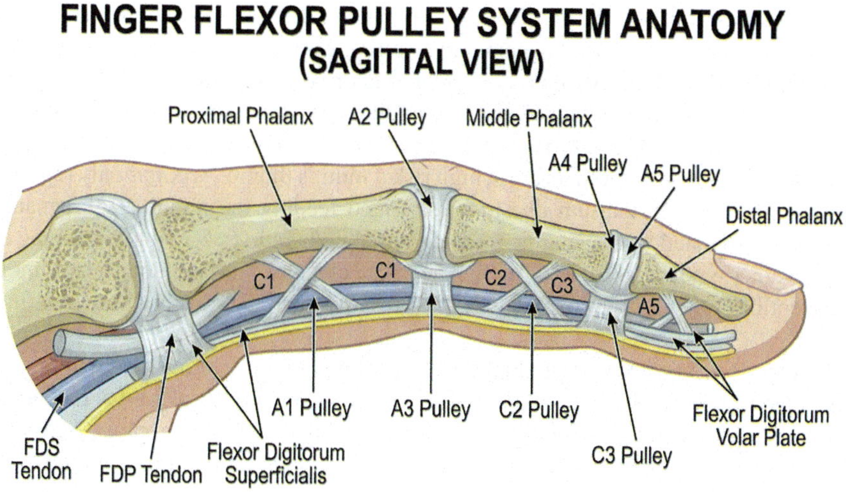

Fig. 6.2 Flexor pulley system of the fingers (sagittal view of a finger showing A1–A5 annular pulleys and cruciform pulleys)

The major peripheral nerves in the hand are the median, ulnar and radial nerves [5]. The median nerve (C6–T1 fibres) travels through the carpal tunnel to supply sensation to the palmar thumb, index, middle and radial half of the ring finger. It also innervates the thenar muscle group (thumb opposition) and the first two lumbricals. The ulnar nerve (C8–T1) passes superficial to the flexor retinaculum (through Guyon's canal) to supply sensation to the ulnar half of the ring and little fingers and motor to the interossei and ulnar lumbricals. Guyon's (ulnar) canal at the wrist lies between the hook of the hamate and pisiform; compression here causes ulnar tunnel syndrome [6]. The radial nerve supplies the dorsal aspect of the hand (thumb side) and the extensor compartments. Its deep branch (posterior interosseous nerve, PIN) winds around the radial head and can be entrapped under the arcade of Frohse (proximal supinator) in the forearm, causing "radial tunnel syndrome" with lateral forearm pain [7].

The wrist allows flexion-extension and radial-ulnar deviation, while forearm pronation-supination occurs at the radioulnar joints. Coordination of these movements requires intact bony alignment, ligament support and smoothly gliding tendons. Understanding this anatomy helps localise pathology based on pain location (e.g. distal radial pain, first compartment or scaphoid; ulnar wrist pain, TFCC or ulnar nerve).

Common Soft Tissue Conditions

De Quervain's Tenosynovitis

De Quervain's tenosynovitis is a stenosing tendinopathy of the first extensor compartment. It involves noninflammatory degeneration (myxoid degeneration) of the tendon sheath of the APL and EPB as they pass under a fibroosseous tunnel at the radial styloid [8]. This causes pain and swelling over the radial wrist, exacerbated by thumb movements. Women are affected approximately four times more often than men [8], and the incidence peaks in middle age. Repetitive use of the thumb in abduction/extension (e.g. lifting a baby, needlework, racquet sports) is a classic precipitant. Indeed, new mothers are at high risk: "mum's thumb" is commonly reported in the first year postpartum due to holding and feeding the infant [9]. Pregnancy itself is associated with a significantly increased odds ratio ($\approx$5.1) for developing de Quervain's syndrome [9], as hormonal and fluid changes make tendon sheaths more susceptible. Other risk factors include diabetes, rheumatoid arthritis and wrist injury.

History Patients describe gradual-onset radial wrist pain, often worse with pinching or grasping an object with the thumb. There is typically focal pain at the lateral wrist just proximal to the thumb base, possibly with swelling or crepitus. Activities involving thumb abduction/extension, pinching, gripping or combined thumb loading with wrist ulnar deviation can precipitate pain. Pain may radiate proximally towards the forearm or distally into the thumb, but there is no numbness (no nerve compression in this tendinopathy). Inflammation is usually limited to the tendon sheath, so systemic symptoms (fever, malaise) are absent unless another inflammatory disorder is present.

Physical Exam Inspection may reveal a tender swelling or nodule at the radial styloid. Palpation of the first dorsal compartment reproduces pain. Range of motion is otherwise normal, and strength testing often shows pain on resisted thumb abduction and extension. A positive Finkelstein's test is often diagnostic: the patient flexes the thumb into the palm and then bends the wrist ulnarly (or the examiner does so)—if this manoeuvre produces sharp pain at the radial styloid, the test is positive [8] (the classic Eichhoff's test variant—making a thumb-in-fist and ulnar deviating—can yield false positives and is less specific). There is no sensory loss, which helps rule out cervical radiculopathy or carpal tunnel. Scaphoid tenderness and ligament testing should be done to exclude bony injury. By contrast, tenderness 4–5 cm more proximally suggests intersection syndrome (inflammation of APL/EPB crossing with extensor carpi radialis), not true De Quervain's [10].

Differential Radial wrist pain can also be caused by intersection syndrome [10] (more dorsally located), osteoarthritis at the thumb carpometacarpal joint or ganglion cysts. In RA, tenosynovitis of multiple compartments can occur, so consider an underlying inflammatory polyarthritis if multiple sites are involved. In gout/pseudogout, acute wrist pain/swelling may mimic tendinitis but is usually more inflammatory with possible systemic signs. Mechanical tendinitis is characterised by activity-related pain that improves with rest, whereas an inflammatory arthritis would have morning stiffness and improvement with use. In De Quervain's, the clear activity link (thumb use) and absence of joint swelling point to a localised tendinopathy rather than diffuse synovitis.

Diagnosis De Quervain's is usually diagnosed clinically. Imaging is often unnecessary unless diagnosis is uncertain. Ultrasound can confirm thickening of the sheath in the first dorsal compartment and allow dynamic testing of tendon gliding. Power Doppler on ultrasound may show hypervascularity in the sheath. X-rays are rarely needed unless fracture is suspected [8]. On occasion, an ultrasound-guided injection of local anaesthetic and corticosteroid may support the diagnosis if it produces clear short-term pain relief, while also providing treatment. Nerve conduction studies are not indicated, since there is no neuropathy.

Trigger Finger (Stenosing Flexor Tenosynovitis)

Trigger finger is a stenosing tenosynovitis of the flexor tendons, typically at the level of the A1 pulley of a finger or thumb (the A1 pulley lies at the base of each finger near the palm). The tendon (often the flexor digitorum superficialis or profundus) develops thickening or a nodule, and the A1 pulley thickens as well, creating a mismatch that catches the tendon during flexion/extension. Patients experience painful locking or catching of the digit: they may have to use the other hand to extend the finger because it is "stuck" in flexion. Most often the ring finger and thumb are involved, but any digit can be affected [11]. The prevalence is about 2% in the general population, peaking in the fifth and sixth decades [11]. Women are more often affected. There is a known association with diabetes mellitus, rheumatoid arthritis, hypothyroidism and other metabolic conditions; for example, systemic "thickening disorders" like diabetes can predispose to pulley/tendon hypertrophy. However, most cases are idiopathic or follow repetitive hand use (e.g. occupational gripping).

History Patients report that one finger (or thumb) intermittently locks or catches when bending or straightening. Early on there may be only clicking or pain in the palm at the base of the finger, but later the finger can "stick" and require manual correction. Pain is usually dull and localised to the palmar aspect of the proximal phalanx/MCP region. There is no numbness or neurological symptoms. Any work or hobby involving repeated gripping or pinching (tools, musical instruments, crafting) may precipitate or worsen symptoms. Tenderness is often present over the involved A1 pulley. Catching may be painless in some chronic cases, but many patients describe pain or tenderness at the A1 pulley, particularly early in the condition. In an acute flexor sheath infection (pyogenic flexor tenosynovitis), there would be fusiform swelling, intense pain even at rest and systemic signs, which is different.

Physical Exam Palpation reveals a tender nodule or thickened flexor tendon sheath at the base of the affected finger. When the examiner moves the finger from extension to flexion, a palpable or audible "pop" may occur as the tendon releases under the pulley. In a full trigger, the finger will lock in flexion and then release with a snap. If held in the locked position, an audible click may occur when it finally extends. One can often reproduce the click by manually flexing and extending the finger while palpating the A1 area. Unlike Dupuytren's contracture, there is no fixed flexion contracture (unless very chronic). Differential includes other causes of finger locking (e.g. extensor tendon subluxation, joint contractures), but trigger finger is usually apparent with a positive palpable triggering on exam.

Diagnosis Clinical. No special imaging is required. Ultrasound may show tendon enlargement or a hypoechoic nodule in the tendon adjacent to the pulley but rarely needed. X-ray is unhelpful. In atypical cases, consider nerve compression (e.g. ulnar nerve if ring/little finger) or basal joint arthritis (grind test of thumb) if thumb triggering could be arthritis-related.

Carpal Tunnel Syndrome (Median Neuropathy at the Wrist)

Carpal tunnel syndrome (CTS) is the most common entrapment neuropathy, caused by compression of the median nerve under the transverse carpal ligament [12].

Typical patients are middle-aged women, although men can also be affected. Known risk factors include diabetes mellitus, hypothyroidism, pregnancy, rheumatoid arthritis and obesity [13]. CTS is especially common in occupations with repetitive wrist/finger use, forceful grip or prolonged wrist flexion/extension (e.g. typing, assembly line work) and can co-occur with pregnancy (fluid retention) or wrist fracture/sprain. It is also often bilateral.

History The cardinal symptoms are numbness, tingling and burning pain in the radial 3½ digits (thumb, index, middle and radial half of ring finger). Symptoms may come and go initially, often worse at night or waking the patient (due to wrist flexion in sleep increasing pressure). Patients may shake or flick their wrist to get relief. As CTS progresses, symptoms can occur during day activities, especially when holding objects (e.g. a phone, steering wheel). Severe cases report weakness or clumsiness of the hand: dropping objects, difficulty with fine manipulation or in chronic advanced cases atrophy of the thenar muscles. Carpal tunnel pain may radiate into the forearm but not above the elbow. Systemic constitutional symptoms are not caused by CTS; however, concurrent fibromyalgia or diabetes may contribute to broader symptoms.

Physical Exam Inspect for thenar eminence wasting. Sensation is tested over the median nerve territory: there may be diminished light touch or two-point discrimination in the index and middle fingers. Tinel's sign (tapping over the median nerve at the wrist) may reproduce tingling in those fingers. Phalen's test (flexing the wrists fully for 30–60 s) often provokes numbness/tingling. Durkan's compression test (firmly pressing on the carpal tunnel for 30 s) can also trigger symptoms. Motor exam may show weak thumb abduction/opposition if severe. Importantly, test the entire upper limb to exclude cervical radiculopathy (C6–C7), brachial plexopathy or proximal median neuropathy (pronator syndrome). Reflexes are normal. The absence of sensory loss or reflex changes (e.g. brachioradialis reflex normal) points away from spinal or central causes.

Diagnosis Initially clinical, but often confirmed by testing. Electrodiagnostic nerve conduction studies (NCS) typically show slowed median sensory and motor latency across the wrist. However, NCS can be negative in very mild cases or early disease, and false positives/negatives occur. Imaging studies may be useful adjuncts. High-resolution ultrasound of the median nerve is increasingly used: it can demonstrate nerve enlargement (increased cross-sectional area) just proximal to the tunnel and flattening within the tunnel [14]. MRI can also show flattening of the nerve and thickening of flexor tendon sheaths but is rarely needed. In practice, a combination of history, exam and NCS is used to confirm CTS. If the diagnosis remains uncertain, nerve conduction is recommended; if NCS is contraindicated or equivocal, ultrasound can be an alternative [15].

Other Entrapment Syndromes

- *Ulnar (Guyon's canal) syndrome*: This is entrapment of the ulnar nerve at the wrist (in Guyon's canal between pisiform and hamate) [6]. It is less common than CTS. Causes include ganglion cysts, bone fractures (hamate hook), anomalous muscles or vascular anomalies and chronic pressure (cyclist's palsy). Patients may have numbness/tingling in the little and ulnar ring finger and weakness of ulnar-innervated intrinsic hand muscles (interossei). Dorsal ulnar hand sensation is typically spared in Guyon's canal syndrome, because the dorsal ulnar cutaneous branch arises proximal to the canal; this can help distinguish it from a more proximal ulnar neuropathy. Examination shows sensory loss on the palmar little finger and weakness of finger abduction/adduction. Palpation might reveal a mass (e.g. ganglion) at the ulnar canal. Diagnosis can be confirmed by EMG/NCS focusing on the distal ulnar nerve or MRI/ultrasound to identify a compressing lesion.
- *Radial tunnel (posterior interosseous) syndrome*: This is entrapment of the deep branch of the radial nerve (posterior interosseous nerve, PIN) in the proximal forearm, often under the supinator. Patients complain of lateral (radial) forearm or elbow pain, often exacerbated by forearm rotation and finger/wrist extension. Unlike CTS, there is typically no sensory loss (the PIN is a motor branch) [7]. On exam, tenderness is usually found 3–5 cm distal to the lateral epicondyle. Wrist and finger extension strength is intact unless the entrapment is advanced (then finger extension weak). Importantly, there is no numbness, distinguishing it from radial sensory neuropathy. This syndrome can be confused with lateral epicondylitis (tennis elbow), since both cause lateral elbow pain. However, resistance testing of finger extension (especially middle finger) is more painful in radial tunnel syndrome. Conservative management (activity modification, NSAIDs, splinting) is first line, but surgery (release of the supinator arch) is indicated if refractory.
- *Thoracic outlet syndrome*: Though not a "hand/wrist" issue, compression of the lower brachial plexus at the thoracic outlet can cause hand numbness; it may cause symptoms in the ulnar-sided hand and forearm, often associated with neck/shoulder posture or arm position; vascular features such as colour change, swelling or altered pulses should be sought.

Mechanical Versus Inflammatory Pain in the Wrist/Hand

It is important to distinguish purely mechanical or overuse pain from pain due to an inflammatory arthritis. Mechanical pain (e.g. tendinitis, nerve entrapment, osteoarthritis) is usually aggravated by activity and relieved by rest; it may worsen towards the end of the day. For example, a worker with early carpal tunnel may notice hand numbness only after hours of typing, and thumb/wrist pain from De Quervain's intensifies with repetitive lifting. Mechanical pain usually lacks systemic features. In contrast, inflammatory pain (e.g. rheumatoid arthritis, crystal arthritis) often features morning stiffness (lasting >30 min) that improves with use, associated with swelling, warmth or systemic symptoms. Patients may describe pain waking them at night or worse upon first awakening. A history of other joint arthritis, rash (psoriasis) or infection (reactive arthritis) should raise suspicion. Laboratory tests (RF, anti-CCP, uric acid, inflammatory markers) and imaging (joint erosions on X-ray, joint effusions on ultrasound/MRI) help confirm inflammatory aetiology.

The clinical exam can also differentiate: inflammatory arthritis often causes symmetric joint swelling and deformities (e.g. rheumatoid swan-neck fingers), whereas a tendinopathy or entrapment causes point tenderness and perhaps crepitus without significant joint effusion. For example, persistent rheumatoid tenosynovitis can mimic De Quervain's but would likely have synovitis elsewhere and positive serologies. In practice, if a patient's hand pain is focal and activity-related with minimal morning stiffness, a mechanical tendon or nerve issue is likely; if there is prolonged morning stiffness, migratory pain or multiple joints involved, investigate inflammatory arthritis.

History and Physical Examination

A thorough history is essential. Questions should characterise *timing* (e.g. insidious vs sudden onset), *aggravating/alleviating* factors (worse with activity vs rest), *associated systemic symptoms* (fever, rash, muscle ache) and *hand usage*. Patients should point to the most painful area—ask the patient to point with one finger to the site of maximal pain, as precise localisation can be very helpful. Ask about occupational/recreational activities involving the hands (keyboarding, sports, instrument playing, knitting, baby care). A history of recent viral illness or infection is relevant (postviral neuritis or arthritis), as is any history of fractures or injections. Enquire about past or family history of rheumatologic disease (RA, lupus, scleroderma, gout). Note risk factors for neuropathy: diabetes, thyroid disease, autoimmune disease or pregnancy. Also ask specifically about any neck or shoulder pain, since cervical radiculopathy or brachial plexus compression can refer symptoms to the hand.

During the physical exam, inspect the entire upper limb. Check for joint effusions, erythema or deformities in the wrist, hand, fingers and neighbouring joints (elbow, shoulder). Assess hand posture: is the thumb held protectively, is there swelling, deformity, triggering or obvious instability? Observe any muscle atrophy (thenar or interossei). Palpate bony landmarks: radial and ulnar styloids, carpal bones and metacarpals. Tenderness localised to a specific tendon sheath or nerve distribution narrows diagnosis, for example, tenderness at the radial styloid (De Quervain's), at the fibrous flexor pulley (trigger finger) or at Guyon's canal (ulnar nerve) vs the carpal tunnel. Perform range of motion for wrist flexion/extension and forearm pronation/supination. Look for crepitus in tendon sheaths (crepitus over the radial wrist suggests intersection syndrome vs De Quervain's).

Neurological Exam Evaluate sensory function in the hand. Check median, ulnar and radial nerve territories (light touch or pinprick on palmar and dorsal aspects). Test motor function of specific muscles: ask the patient to abduct/adduct fingers (ulnar nerve interossei), oppose the thumb (median nerve) and extend the wrist and fingers (radial nerve). Evaluate reflexes (biceps, triceps, brachioradialis) to screen for proximal pathology. Distinguish peripheral nerve findings from spinal cord/radicular signs: for example, if you suspect carpal tunnel, also ensure cervical spine exam and Spurling's test are normal to exclude C6–C7 radiculopathy.

Special Tests A variety of provocative manoeuvres help identify specific syndromes:

- *Finkelstein's test (De Quervain's)*: Patient makes a fist with thumb inside the fingers, or examiner grasps patient's thumb. The wrist is then passively ulnarly deviated. A positive test reproduces pain at the radial styloid, confirming first compartment tenosynovitis.
- *Phalen's manoeuvre (carpal tunnel)*: Have the patient hold both wrists in flexion (back of hands together) for 30–60 s. Tingling or numbness in the median nerve distribution indicates a positive sign.
- *Tinel's sign (median nerve at wrist)*: Lightly tap the volar wrist over the carpal tunnel. Tingling in the thumb/index/middle fingers within seconds suggests median nerve irritability.
- *Durkan's (compression) test*: Firm pressure over the carpal tunnel for 30 s; reproduction of symptoms is positive.
- *Thumb grind test*: Press and rotate the thumb metacarpal into the trapezium. Pain suggests thumb carpometacarpal osteoarthritis, which can mimic trigger thumb symptoms.
- *Lunate/scapholunate (Watson) tests*: These help identify carpal bone instability, not the focus of this chapter.
- *Grip strength and pinch*: Assess for weakness. For carpal tunnel syndrome, assess thumb abduction and opposition; for ulnar nerve dysfunction, assess finger abduction/adduction and key pinch.

It is important to interpret special tests in context: for example, Finkelstein's is very sensitive for De Quervain's but should be done carefully to avoid false positives from other radial wrist pain. Phalen's and Tinel's tests are not perfectly specific or sensitive (some studies show Phalen's ~50–85% sensitive) [16], so they are most useful combined with the clinical picture and, if needed, confirmatory studies.

Diagnostic Tools

- *Plain radiographs*: X-rays of the wrist/hand are often obtained to rule out fractures, arthritis or mass lesions in unexplained cases. They have limited utility for soft tissue disorders: they do not show tendon changes. They can, however, detect bony causes of pain (e.g. hook of hamate fracture in ulnar neuropathy).
- *Ultrasound:* Musculoskeletal ultrasound is excellent for visualising tendons, pulleys and nerves. It can detect thickening of tendon sheaths in De Quervain's

or trigger finger. For CTS, ultrasound can visualise median nerve enlargement (cross-sectional area) and the "flattening" at the entrance to the carpal tunnel. High-resolution dynamic ultrasound can also guide injections into tendon sheaths or the carpal tunnel with precise needle placement (improving outcomes). Ultrasound is low cost and quick and does not require contrast or radiation, making it a useful first-line imaging modality for unexplained hand pain.

- *Electrodiagnostic studies:* Nerve conduction studies (NCS) and electromyography (EMG) remain the diagnostic gold standard for neuropathies. In CTS, slowing of median nerve conduction velocity across the wrist and delayed distal motor latency are diagnostic. EMG can show denervation in severe cases. However, NCS/EMG are operator-dependent and may be uncomfortable; they can be falsely negative in mild CTS [17]. In suspected ulnar or radial tunnel syndromes, EMG may confirm conduction block or rule out proximal issues. In practice, mild cases of CTS can be managed initially without NCS; if symptoms persist or are atypical, NCS/EMG should be done to confirm the diagnosis.
- *MRI:* MRI of the wrist or hand provides detailed soft tissue contrast. It can detect tenosynovial inflammation, tendon tears and nerve compression. For example, MRI may show thickened flexor tendon sheaths or bowstringing in trigger finger or median nerve compression in CTS. MRI is expensive and static (cannot do dynamic tests), so it is reserved for cases where ultrasound and NCS are inconclusive or when space-occupying lesions (tumours, anomalous muscles) are suspected.

Laboratory tests are not usually needed for pure mechanical tendinopathies. However, if an underlying inflammatory condition is suspected (e.g. rheumatoid arthritis causing tenosynovitis), appropriate blood tests (RF, anti-CCP, ESR/CRP, urate level) should be ordered. A synovial or tendon sheath fluid aspiration may be considered if infection or crystal disease is a concern.

Management

Conservative Therapy

Initial management of hand/wrist tendinopathies and mild nerve entrapments is usually nonsurgical. The principles include resting the affected area, reducing aggravating activities and using supportive devices and medications to decrease inflammation and pain.

- *Splinting/bracing*: Immobilisation allows irritated tendons or nerves to heal. For De Quervain's, a thumb spica splint (immobilising the thumb and wrist in a neutral or slight extension position) is worn, typically for 4–6 weeks [4]. This offloads the first compartment and relieves pain. For trigger finger, a stiff digital splint blocking the involved joint (usually the proximal interphalangeal joint) can prevent triggering and allow rest. In early CTS, a neutral-position wrist splint at night can prevent flexion stress on the nerve and reduce nocturnal symptoms. Prolonged use of a splint helps break the pain cycle while other therapies are tried.

- *Activity modification*: Identify and temporarily avoid the actions that provoke symptoms. For a new mother with De Quervain's, this may mean minimising lifting the baby or altering the way she holds the infant (supporting the hand/wrist differently). Computer users with CTS should take frequent breaks, correct ergonomics and avoid extreme wrist postures. Even simple adjustments (e.g. using a lighter grip, powering nail guns with straps, wearing padded gloves) can reduce tendon stress. Education on proper technique (such as lifting with more of the whole hand rather than pinching with the thumb alone) is vital.
- *Nonsteroidal antiinflammatory drugs (NSAIDs)*: For mechanical tendinopathies, NSAIDs (ibuprofen, naproxen, etc.) can ease pain, particularly in the acute phase. They may reduce the secondary inflammation of the sheath. For example, patients with De Quervain's are often advised to take NSAIDs to control pain. In CTS, systemic NSAIDs have limited long-term benefit (the underlying pathology is a fixed compression), but a short course can help with associated tenosynovitis.
- *Physiotherapy/occupational therapy*: A therapist can teach stretching and strengthening exercises for the hand and wrist. For De Quervain's, gentle stretching of the thumb tendons and thumb-strengthening exercises can improve tendon gliding. For CTS, exercises to mobilise the median nerve (nerve glides) and to strengthen wrist/arm muscles may help. Soft tissue mobilisation and gentle tendon gliding techniques are often used. Therapists also advise on ergonomic changes and activity pacing.
- *Ultrasound-guided hydrodissection*: A newer conservative technique for entrapment—injecting saline or lidocaine under ultrasound guidance around an entrapped nerve to mechanically separate it from surrounding tissue. One study showed steroid injections provided significant relief in ~95% of De Quervain's patients [18]. Similarly, for carpal tunnel, hydrodissection of the median nerve combined with steroid injection has been reported to improve symptoms [19]. However, these techniques should be performed by experienced providers and evidence is still evolving.
- *Observation*: Mild cases, especially in pregnancy/postpartum, may improve spontaneously as fluid balance normalises or as the patient adapts her activities. A period of watchful waiting with conservative care is reasonable if symptoms are mild and function is preserved.

Injection Therapy

Corticosteroid injections are a mainstay for many refractory or moderate cases, particularly for De Quervain's, trigger finger and sometimes CTS. The steroid reduces tendon sheath inflammation and swelling, often dramatically relieving pain for months.

- *De Quervain's*: A local injection of corticosteroid into the first dorsal compartment can significantly improve symptoms. Ultrasound guidance is recommended if available, because it ensures accurate delivery into the tendon sheath space. A recent systematic review found that ultrasound-guided steroid injections achieved complete symptom resolution in about 74% of wrists [18], significantly better than blind injections. Pain scores were lower and recurrence rates were fewer with ultrasound guidance. Often only one or two injections are needed, although symptoms can recur in some. Postinjection, patients should rest the thumb for a few days and continue splinting briefly.
- *Trigger finger*: Steroid injection into the flexor tendon sheath at the A1 pulley is effective in many cases. Randomised trials have shown corticosteroids outperform saline placebo [11]. Typically, a single injection relieves triggering in about 50–80% of patients (some studies report around two-thirds of fingers improved) [11]. Diabetic patients and multiple-digit cases may have lower success. Injections can often be done blind (by palpating the pulley), but ultrasound guidance can improve accuracy and reduce inadvertent intratendinous injection. Side effects are rare but can include short-lived swelling or tendon weakening.
- *Carpal tunnel syndrome*: Local corticosteroid injection into the carpal tunnel can provide temporary relief, especially in mild to moderate cases. Injections may improve symptoms for several weeks to months, but long-term cure is unlikely without addressing the compression. Many clinicians reserve this for patients who are not surgical candidates or as a temporising measure. (Large trials have compared injection vs night splints, showing equivalent short-term relief [20].) Repeat injections are possible but repeated steroid can atrophy fat or tendon and risk infection. Notably, splinting and corticosteroid injection generally have low rates of serious adverse events compared with surgery, although recurrence is common.
- *Other tenosynovitis*: Steroid injections into other inflamed tendon sheaths (e.g. extensor carpi ulnaris, biceps) can be done similarly, though careful localisation is needed.

Ultrasound-guided ganglion cyst aspiration/injection (with steroid) is an option for space-occupying causes. Hyaluronic acid injections into tendons have been explored (especially in trigger finger) but have not shown clear superiority to steroids [21]. Platelet-rich plasma (PRP) injections are under investigation for hand and wrist tendinopathies but are not standard in rheumatology practice just yet.

Indications for Surgical Referral

When conservative measures fail or if there is progressive neurologic compromise, surgical intervention is indicated.

- *De Quervain's*: If 8–12 weeks of conservative therapy (splint, NSAIDs, injection) fails to relieve severe symptoms, surgical release is considered. The procedure (first dorsal compartment release) involves opening the sheath longitudinally to free the APL/EPB tendons. This is an outpatient minor surgery. Postsurgery therapy focuses on thumb mobilisation and gradual return to activity. Most patients improve, though wound pain and scar sensitivity may persist for weeks. Rarely, nerve branches (superficial radial nerve) can be irritated during surgery causing sensory changes.

- *Trigger finger*: Surgery (A1 pulley release) is recommended for fingers that remain locked despite injections or for severe triggering (e.g. thumb triggering that impairs gripping). The release can be done percutaneously or with a small open incision, cutting the pulley. Success rates exceed 90% and complications are low (minor scar pain, rarely tendon bowstringing). If bilateral or multiple fingers are affected, each finger is treated separately.
- *Carpal tunnel syndrome*: Surgical decompression is indicated for moderate-to-severe CTS or any case with constant numbness, muscle weakness/atrophy or failure to improve after conservative care. Typically, if a patient has ongoing night-time numbness after 2–3 months of splinting/injection, surgery is offered. Endoscopic or open carpal tunnel release has excellent success (>90% good outcome) with minimal risk. Preoperative nerve studies and ultrasound can confirm diagnosis and severity; after surgery, therapy is minimal and return to work is usually within weeks. High-risk patients (diabetics, rheumatoid arthritis) may have slower recovery.
- *Ulnar nerve (Guyon's)*: Rarely, if a clear compressive lesion (cyst, tumour, anomalous muscle) is identified, surgical decompression is done. Work-related mild ulnar neuropathies (e.g. handlebar palsy) usually improve with padding and behaviour change; persistent cases may need surgical decompression of the canal.
- *Radial tunnel*: Surgery (radial tunnel release) is considered only after extensive nonsurgical treatment (at least 6 months) has failed, due to variable outcomes.

In general, surgical referrals are made when diagnostic certainty is high and the impairment is significant. Comanagement with hand surgery specialists is common in rheumatology practice for these procedures.

Prognosis and Outcomes

Prognosis is generally good with proper treatment but varies by condition and patient factors. Many tendinopathies improve with conservative care:

- *De Quervain's*: With early treatment, many patients resolve with splinting and NSAIDs. When given steroid injection, over 70% have complete resolution of symptoms [18], and most others have at least partial relief. If surgery is done, most will have lasting relief, though some may have minor residual tenderness. Recurrence after surgery is rare. Long-term function is usually normal; untreated chronic cases can lead to persistent discomfort and compensatory wrist movement.

- *Trigger finger*: Approximately 50–90% of cases respond to a single steroid injection (higher if treated early) [11]. Diabetics respond less well. Some will need a second injection; overall, 60–70% may avoid surgery with injection therapy alone. Surgery has a very high success (nearly 100% resolution of triggering), so even refractory cases do well. Patients may experience local pain/bruising after injection or scar tenderness after surgery, but return to full function is expected.
- *Carpal tunnel syndrome*: Mild cases can be managed conservatively for years with splints and lifestyle adjustments. In moderate cases, steroid injection often provides months of relief, but long-term recurrence is common (many patients opt for surgery eventually). In severe CTS (muscle atrophy or constant numbness), prompt surgical release is usually necessary. Surgical outcome is generally excellent: most patients have improvement in numbness and strength; however, full recovery of numbness may take months [22]. Some patients have persistent dysesthesia due to chronic nerve damage. Diabetes and long-standing symptoms predict a slower or incomplete recovery.
- *Ulnar (Guyon) and radial tunnel*: Data are limited. Conservative management often resolves mild cases over months. Surgical decompression of Guyon canal cysts or radial tunnel has mixed success (~50–80% improve) and carries risk of nerve injury, so it is reserved for severe, clearly defined cases.

Overall, key prognostic factors include duration of symptoms (chronicity worsens prognosis), severity at presentation (constant numbness or weakness suggests more nerve damage), and associated conditions (diabetes and rheumatoid arthritis are associated with recurrence or slower healing). Patient education on activity modification is crucial to prevent recurrence after initial therapy.

Key Learning Points

- De Quervain's tenosynovitis is a non-inflammatory stenosing tendinopathy/tenosynovial disorder of the first dorsal compartment involving APL and EPB, causing radial wrist pain. It is common postpartum or after repetitive thumb use.
- Finkelstein's test is diagnostic. Initial treatment: thumb spica splint, NSAIDs, then steroid injection if needed. Surgery if refractory.
- Trigger finger (stenosing flexor tenosynovitis) usually involves the A1 pulley at the base of a finger. Patients present with locking/clicking of a digit. Conservative care (finger splint, activity change) and corticosteroid injection can resolve most cases; surgery (A1 release) is curative if needed.
- Carpal tunnel syndrome (CTS) is median nerve compression under the flexor retinaculum. Symptoms: nocturnal numbness in thumb/index/middle fingers. Exam: Tinel's and Phalen's tests. Confirm with nerve conduction studies or ultrasound. Treat mild CTS with wrist splinting at night, NSAIDs and corticosteroid injection; refer severe or refractory cases for surgical release.
- Differentiate mechanical vs inflammatory causes of wrist pain by history: mechanical pain is use-related and end-of-day; inflammatory pain has morning

stiffness and systemic features. Always consider rheumatoid arthritis, gout or polymyalgia rheumatica in the differential of chronic hand/wrist pain.

- History and exam are most important. Localise the pain (e.g. radial styloid, De Quervain's; palmar base of finger, trigger finger; carpal tunnel distribution, CTS). Perform special tests (Finkelstein's, Tinel's, Phalen's). Assess for tendon vs joint vs nerve pathology. Use imaging (ultrasound, MRI) and electrodiagnostics (EMG/NCS) to confirm uncertain cases.
- Conservative management (splinting, activity modification, physiotherapy and NSAIDs) is first line. Corticosteroid injection is highly effective for tenosynovitis. Ultrasound guidance improves injection accuracy and outcomes. Hydrodissection is an emerging technique for nerve entrapment.
- Indications for surgery include locked or refractory trigger finger, persistent median nerve dysfunction despite conservative care or structural lesions. Surgical release of pulleys or the transverse carpal ligament is generally safe and effective when indicated.
- Prognosis is generally excellent with timely treatment. Recurrence can occur (e.g. after steroid injection) but repeat injection or surgery can address it. Chronic untreated tendon entrapment may lead to permanent limitation, so early diagnosis and management are important.

References

1. Erwin J, Varacallo MA. Anatomy, shoulder and upper limb, wrist joint. StatPearls; 2026. Available from: http://www.ncbi.nlm.nih.gov/pubmed/7408322.
2. Doyle JR. Anatomy of the flexor tendon sheath and pulley system: a current review. J Hand Surg Am. 1989;14(2 Pt 2):349–51. Available from: http://www.ncbi.nlm.nih.gov/pubmed/2732428.
3. Jeanmonod R, Tiwari V, Waseem M. Trigger Finger. StatPearls; 2026. Available from: http://www.ncbi.nlm.nih.gov/pubmed/30676573.
4. Satteson E, Tannan SC. De Quervain tenosynovitis. StatPearls; 2026. Available from: http://www.ncbi.nlm.nih.gov/pubmed/34506345.
5. Matloub HS, Yousif NJ. Peripheral nerve anatomy and innervation pattern. Hand Clin. 1992;8(2):201–14. Available from: http://www.ncbi.nlm.nih.gov/pubmed/1613029.
6. Aleksenko D, Varacallo MA. Guyon Canal syndrome. StatPearls; 2026. Available from: http://www.ncbi.nlm.nih.gov/pubmed/28594495.
7. Shamrock AG, Das JM. Radial tunnel syndrome. StatPearls; 2026. Available from: http://www.ncbi.nlm.nih.gov/pubmed/19969199.
8. Som A, Wermuth HR, Singh P. Finkelstein sign. StatPearls; 2026. Available from: http://www.ncbi.nlm.nih.gov/pubmed/18063716.
9. Smith GB, Young B, Titan AL, Kenney DE, Ladd AL. Incidence and risk factors for soft tissue hand and wrist conditions in pregnancy and postpartum. J Hand Surg Glob. 2025;7(5):100778. Available from: http://www.ncbi.nlm.nih.gov/pubmed/40746749.
10. Skinner TM. Intersection syndrome: the subtle squeak of an overused wrist. J Am Board Fam Med. 2017;30(4):547–51. Available from: http://www.ncbi.nlm.nih.gov/pubmed/28720637.
11. Donati D, Ricci V, Boccolari P, Origlio F, Vita F, Naňka O, et al. From diagnosis to rehabilitation of trigger finger: a narrative review. BMC Musculoskelet Disord. 2024;25(1):1061. Available from: https://bmcmusculoskeletdisord.biomedcentral.com/articles/10.1186/s12891-024-08192-5.

12. Kim P-T, Lee H-J, Kim T-G, Jeon I-H. Current approaches for carpal tunnel syndrome. Clin Orthop Surg. 2014;6(3):253–7. Available from: http://www.ncbi.nlm.nih.gov/pubmed/25177448.
13. Karne SS, Bhalerao NS. Carpal tunnel syndrome in hypothyroidism. J Clin Diagn Res. 2016;10(2):OC36-8. Available from: http://www.ncbi.nlm.nih.gov/pubmed/27042500.
14. Tomažin T, Pušnik L, Albano D, Jengojan SA, Snoj Ž. Multiparametric ultrasound assessment of carpal tunnel syndrome: beyond nerve cross-sectional area. Semin Musculoskelet Radiol. 2024;28(6):661–71. Available from: http://www.ncbi.nlm.nih.gov/pubmed/39561748.
15. Azami A, Maleki N, Anari H, Iranparvar Alamdari M, Kalantarhormozi M, Tavosi Z. The diagnostic value of ultrasound compared with nerve conduction velocity in carpal tunnel syndrome. Int J Rheum Dis. 2014;17(6):612–20. Available from: http://www.ncbi.nlm.nih.gov/pubmed/24618125.
16. Wiesman IM, Novak CB, Mackinnon SE, Winograd JM. Sensitivity and specificity of clinical testing for carpal tunnel syndrome. Can J Plast Surg. 2003;11(2):70–2. Available from: http://www.ncbi.nlm.nih.gov/pubmed/24222987.
17. Zaki HA, Shaban E, Salem W, Bilal F, Fayed M, Hendy M, et al. A comparative analysis between ultrasound and Electromyographic and nerve conduction studies in diagnosing carpal tunnel syndrome (CTS): a systematic review and meta-analysis. Cureus. 2022;14(10):e30476. Available from: http://www.ncbi.nlm.nih.gov/pubmed/36415360.
18. He KS, He KS, Cheah A, Al-Halabi B, Danino MA, Efanov JI. Unblinding de Quervain: a systematic review of ultrasound-guided injection of corticosteroids for treatment of stenosing tenosynovitis of the 1st extensor compartment. J Med Radiat Sci. 2023;70(3):319–26. Available from: http://www.ncbi.nlm.nih.gov/pubmed/37078429.
19. Cage ES, Beyer JJ, Ebraheim NA. Injections for treatment of carpal tunnel syndrome: a narrative review of the literature. J Orthop. 2023;37:81–5. Available from: http://www.ncbi.nlm.nih.gov/pubmed/36974095.
20. Burton C, Rathod-Mistry T, Blackburn S, Blagojevic-Bucknall M, Chesterton L, Davenport G, et al. The effectiveness of corticosteroid injection versus night splints for carpal tunnel syndrome: 24-month follow-up of a randomized trial. Rheumatology (Oxford). 2023;62(2):546–54. Available from: http://www.ncbi.nlm.nih.gov/pubmed/35394019.
21. Navaneeth P, Geevarughese NM, Bhat AK. Effectiveness of steroid injection on functional outcomes in adults with trigger finger: a systematic review and meta-analysis protocol. BMJ Open. 2025;15(11):e110059. Available from: https://bmjopen.bmj.com/lookup/doi/10.1136/bmjopen-2025-110059.
22. Alimohammadi E, Bagheri SR, Hadidi H, Rizevandi P, Abdi A. Carpal tunnel surgery: predictors of clinical outcomes and patients' satisfaction. BMC Musculoskelet Disord. 2020;21(1):51. Available from: http://www.ncbi.nlm.nih.gov/pubmed/31992298.

Spine and Axial Soft Tissue Pain

7

Abstract

Spine and axial pain are among the most common reasons for patient visits in rheumatology, sport and exercise medicine and primary care. This chapter reviews the anatomy, common causes and evaluation of axial spine pain, emphasising both mechanical and inflammatory aetiologies. We describe cervical, thoracic and lumbar spinal structures and biomechanics and focus on soft tissue sources of pain such as muscular strain, myofascial trigger points and sacroiliac joint dysfunction. Axial spondyloarthritis includes radiographic disease, historically termed ankylosing spondylitis, and non-radiographic axial spondyloarthritis. This condition is discussed as a classic inflammatory cause, along with distinguishing features of inflammatory vs mechanical back pain. Red flags (infection, malignancy, fracture, cauda equina) are highlighted. We outline key elements of the spine examination, imaging strategies (when to use X-ray, MRI and ultrasound) and relevant laboratory tests (HLA-B27, CRP, ESR) for axial pain. Diagnostic criteria and screening tools for axial spondyloarthritis are reviewed. Management strategies emphasise conservative therapy: patient education, physiotherapy (posture correction, core strengthening) and manual techniques, with trigger point injections reserved for refractory myofascial pain. Pharmacological treatment includes NSAIDs (non-steroidal anti-inflammatory drugs) for both mechanical and inflammatory pain, analgesics as needed and biologic therapies for axial SpA. We discuss criteria for specialist referral and outline rehabilitation principles. Prognosis of axial pain depends on underlying cause. This comprehensive review equips clinicians with a practical approach to spine pain in rheumatologic practice.

© The Author(s), under exclusive license to Springer Nature Switzerland AG 2026

R. Amarnani, *Soft Tissue and Musculoskeletal Medicine in Rheumatology*,
https://doi.org/10.1007/978-3-032-29441-8_7

Clinical Vignette

A 38-year-old man presents with a 6-month history of low back pain radiating to the buttocks. He reports gradual onset of dull pain that is worse after inactivity or on waking but improves with exercise and warm showers. He notes stiffness lasting about 30 minutes each morning and occasional pain awakening him at night. He has no history of trauma or systemic symptoms. On exam, lumbar flexion is limited with discomfort, and there is mild tenderness over the sacroiliac areas bilaterally. Neurologic exam is normal, with intact reflexes and sensation. Initial laboratory tests show an elevated C-reactive protein and a positive HLA-B27. A pelvic X-ray is unremarkable, but sacroiliac MRI demonstrates bone marrow oedema at the SI joints. This presentation is highly suggestive of axial spondyloarthritis; the patient is managed with NSAIDs and referred to a rheumatologist. He also receives physiotherapy focusing on core strengthening and posture correction. Over the following months, his pain improves with therapy and medical management.

Anatomy and Biomechanics of the Cervical, Thoracic and Lumbar Spine

Cervical Spine

The cervical spine (C1–C7) supports the head and allows a wide range of motion. The atlantooccipital joint (C0–C1) and the atlantoaxial joint (C1–C2) permit nodding and rotation, respectively [1]. Cervical vertebral bodies are smaller with thinner intervertebral discs, reflecting lower weight-bearing demands. Unique features include transverse foramina (for vertebral arteries) and bifid spinous processes. The natural cervical lordosis (inward curve) centres the head over the spine. Cervical facets are oriented roughly at 45° to the horizontal, allowing flexion, extension, lateral bending and rotation. Ligaments (tectorial membrane, ligamentum flavum, nuchal ligament) add stability [1].

Thoracic Spine

The thoracic spine (T1–T12) has a natural kyphotic curve (outward). Thoracic vertebrae articulate with ribs at costovertebral joints, forming a rigid rib cage. Facet joints here are more coronally oriented (around 60°) than in the cervical spine, which favours rotation and lateral flexion but limits extension [2]. Long, overlapping spinous processes and the presence of ribs substantially restrict motion. The disc-to-body height ratio is lower than in cervical/lumbar (roughly 1:5), reflecting relative inflexibility. The thoracic region is relatively less mobile than the cervical and lumbar spine, although postural and myofascial pain remain common.

Lumbar Spine and Sacrum

The lumbar spine (L1–L5) is built for maximum weight-bearing. Vertebral bodies are large, with thick intervertebral discs (disc height ~1/3 of vertebral height) that absorb shock. A lumbar lordosis (inward curve) allows upright posture and mobility. Facet joints in the lumbar spine are oriented nearly sagittally (up to ~90°), permitting flexion/extension but resisting rotation [3]. This orientation, combined with stout ligaments (iliolumbar, ligamentum flavum), stabilises the lower spine under load. The sacrum (S1–S5 fused) connects the spine to the pelvis via the sacroiliac joints (SIJs). The SIJs are true diarthrodial joints (synovial anteriorly, syndesmotic posteriorly) with limited motion—they primarily transmit axial load from spine to hips [4].

The spine as a whole distributes axial loads and allows coordinated motion. Vertebral bodies and discs bear most compressive force, especially in the lumbar region. Facet joints guide motion and share extension loads: for example, lumbar flexion increases load on the anterior disc and stretches posterior ligaments, whereas extension compresses the facets [5]. The natural curvatures of the spine act as springs that balance the head and trunk; maintaining normal curvature (with active core muscle engagement) minimises stress. The spinal cord ends near L1–L2 (conus medullaris), and below this level, the cauda equina occupies the canal; this is important for correlating symptoms with imaging. Each functional spinal unit (two vertebrae, disc and facets) provides flexibility and stability, maintained by ligaments and paraspinal muscle tension. The paraspinal muscles provide dynamic control: the erector spinae (iliocostalis, longissimus, spinalis) extend the spine, while deeper muscles (multifidus, rotatores) stabilise each segment (Fig. 7.1).

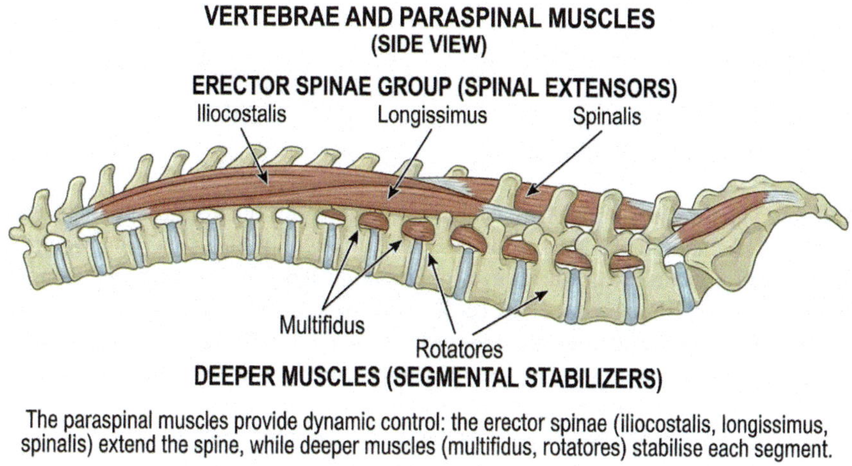

Fig. 7.1 Vertebrae and paraspinal muscle anatomy

Paraspinal Muscles

The extrinsic back muscles (trapezius, latissimus dorsi, levator scapulae) connect the spine to the shoulder girdle and scapula and can contribute to neck/back pain when strained. The intrinsic muscles (superficial layers, splenius capitis/cervicis; intermediate, erector spinae; deep, multifidus, rotatores and interspinales) maintain posture and control small movements [6]. For example, multifidus spans each vertebra and is critical for segmental stabilisation; atrophy or dysfunction can lead to lumbar instability. The thoracolumbar fascia in the lower back transmits forces between trunk and pelvis; it contains proprioceptive and nociceptive fibres and can be a source of pain when injured.

Common Soft Tissue Causes of Spinal Pain

Cervical Strain and Tension-Type Neck Pain

Nonspecific neck pain often stems from muscle strain or tension. Poor posture (forward head, rounded shoulders) or repetitive stress (texting, desk work) tightens the posterior cervical muscles (trapezius, levator scapulae, suboccipital). Patients report localised pain or stiffness that worsens with prolonged head flexion. On exam, there may be tenderness and trigger points in the upper trapezius, reduced range of motion and pain with resisted neck extension. Cervicogenic headache (referred head pain from C1 to C3 structures) can coexist. Acute injuries (whiplash) cause muscle strain and possibly facet joint irritation. Overuse of neck muscles can also lead to tension-type headaches referred from the suboccipital and trapezius areas. Inflammatory or degenerative joint disease (e.g. rheumatoid arthritis, cervical spondylosis) can cause neck pain but those involve structural pathology rather than pure soft tissue pain.

Myofascial Pain Syndromes

Myofascial pain syndrome (MPS) is characterised by discrete trigger points in muscles and associated fascia that produce referred pain. It often arises from repetitive muscle overuse, chronic postural stress or emotional tension. For instance, sustained contraction of the upper trapezius (desk work or stress) can create active trigger points radiating pain into the shoulder or head. In the low back, hypertonic quadratus lumborum or gluteal muscles may develop painful knots that mimic discogenic pain. Patients with MPS usually report constant deep aching pain in the muscle belly or tendon, and pressing on a trigger point can reproduce the pain and even cause twitch in the muscle. MPS pain may not respond well to oral analgesics; instead, physical approaches (stretching, dry needling, massage) targeting the trigger point are more effective. Chronic stress and poor sleep can exacerbate myofascial pain.

Mechanical Low Back Pain

Mechanical low back pain arises from musculoskeletal structures (discs, ligaments, muscles, facets) without systemic inflammation. It is often acute or subacute following an injury or strain. Common sources include lumbar muscle strain/sprain, degenerative disc disease (discogenic pain), facet osteoarthritis and spondylosis with osteophytes [7]. Disc herniation or bulge can irritate nerve roots (radiculopathy), usually causing leg pain. Facet-mediated pain characteristically worsens with lumbar extension and improves with flexion. Degenerative spondylolisthesis or stenosis can cause mechanical neurogenic claudication. In many cases, no single lesion is identified (termed "nonspecific low back pain"). Clinical clues are usually mild: pain occurs with certain movements (lifting, bending, prolonged standing) and improves with rest. There are no systemic symptoms, and laboratory tests/imaging reveal only age-appropriate degenerative changes. Chronic mechanical pain is influenced by deconditioned paraspinal muscles, weak core musculature and psychosocial factors (fear-avoidance behaviour), which all should be addressed in management. Facet arthritis becomes common with age, often causing low back or neck pain that is posture-dependent.

Sacroiliac Joint Dysfunction

Sacroiliac (SI) joint pain is often overlooked but can account for ~25% of chronic low back pain [8]. The pain is usually below the posterior iliac spine, in the buttock, in groin or posterior thigh and is typically unilateral (though it can be bilateral). It tends to worsen with weight-bearing activities (walking, standing), climbing stairs or prolonged sitting. Pregnancy, gait asymmetry or leg length discrepancy can predispose to SIJ stress. On exam, tenderness may be elicited just below the PSIS (Fortin finger sign). Provocative tests (Gaenslen's test, FABER/Patrick's test, thigh thrust, compression, distraction) can reproduce SIJ pain. A cluster (e.g. ≥3 of 5 tests positive) increases diagnostic certainty [9]. Image-guided diagnostic SIJ local anaesthetic block is often considered the reference standard, although it is not routinely required in typical clinical practice. Treatment starts conservatively: pelvic stabilisation exercises and manual therapy. If severe or refractory, image-guided SIJ injections (local anaesthetic + steroid) or radiofrequency ablation of the lateral branches may be considered. Chronic SIJ inflammation (sacroiliitis) can also occur in axial SpA (see below), so coexisting inflammatory features (morning stiffness, HLA-B27) should be noted.

Inflammatory Causes: Axial Spondyloarthritis (axSpA)

Axial spondyloarthritis is a chronic inflammatory arthritis primarily affecting the spine and sacroiliac joints. Ankylosing spondylitis (AS) refers to radiographic axSpA (bilateral sacroiliitis visible on X-ray), while non-radiographic axial spondyloarthritis lacks definite radiographic sacroiliitis but may show active inflammation on MRI, or meet classification through HLA-B27 positivity with SpA features. AxSpA typically presents in younger adults (often <45 years) and is more common in men. The hallmark is chronic inflammatory back pain: insidious onset, morning stiffness, pain often improving with exercise but not with rest and frequent night-time awakening [10]. Patients often report stiffness that eases within an hour of activity. Peripheral enthesitis is common (e.g. Achilles tendonitis, plantar fasciitis pain). About 25–40% of patients experience acute anterior uveitis (eye inflammation) [11]. Other associations include psoriasis, inflammatory bowel disease and peripheral arthritis, with hip and shoulder involvement occurring in some patients.

Laboratory findings: HLA-B27 is positive in ~80–90% of AS patients, greatly increasing disease risk, though it is not diagnostic alone (present in ~7.5% of healthy people, <5% of whom develop AS) [12]. Acute phase reactants (CRP, ESR) may be elevated during active inflammation, but up to half of patients can have normal CRP/ESR despite active disease [13]. Radiographically, early disease shows sacroiliitis (erosion, sclerosis) on pelvis X-ray or bone oedema on MRI, and late AS shows "bamboo spine" (vertebral fusion) and syndesmophytes. MRI STIR sequences are sensitive for early sacroiliac and vertebral inflammation. Recognition of axSpA is critical, as prompt treatment (NSAIDs and biologic agents) can improve symptoms and possibly slow progression.

Differentiation Between Mechanical and Inflammatory Back Pain

Mechanical back pain and inflammatory back pain have distinct clinical patterns. Mechanical pain is usually acute or subacute and activity-related, worsened by bending/lifting and relieved by rest. It does not typically disturb sleep. In contrast, inflammatory back pain (IBP) is chronic (>3 months) and often begins before age 40, with insidious onset, prolonged morning stiffness, pain that improves with movement and nocturnal pain (especially second-half of sleep) [14]. IBP may also be accompanied by other SpA features (enthesitis, arthritis, uveitis). A history of psoriasis, IBD or family history of SpA favours inflammatory causes. If suspicion is low (lacking IBP features, older age, clear mechanical trigger, normal laboratory tests), mechanical causes are presumed. Conversely, red flags or IBP features prompt evaluation for axial SpA or other pathology.

Red Flag Features

Certain findings warrant urgent consideration of serious underlying causes. Key red flags include the following:

- *Neurologic compromise:* Progressive lower extremity weakness, sensory loss or new bowel/bladder dysfunction (suggestive of cauda equina or spinal cord compression).

- *Infection:* Fever, night sweats, immunosuppression, intravenous drug use or recent infection (risk of vertebral osteomyelitis/epidural abscess). Severe back pain and high CRP/ESR raise suspicion.
- *Malignancy:* Personal history of cancer, unexplained weight loss and history of metastasis to bone. Constant night pain not relieved by posture is concerning. Lab clues (hypercalcemia) or abnormal blood counts may appear.
- *Fracture:* Significant trauma or trivial trauma in an older person (osteoporosis), long-term corticosteroid use or severe focal vertebral tenderness.
- *Age extremes:* Back pain before age 20 (juvenile SpA, tumour) or after 55 (spinal stenosis, compression fracture) may indicate pathology.
- *Other:* Cauda equina symptoms (saddle anaesthesia, urinary retention) demand emergency referral.
- Red flags should prompt urgent assessment and appropriately targeted imaging, usually MRI when infection, malignancy, cord compression or cauda equina syndrome is suspected.

Physical Examination of the Spine and Soft Tissues

A complete exam helps localise pain and identify deficits.

Inspection: Note posture (cervical lordosis, thoracic kyphosis, lumbar lordosis), limb length discrepancy, pelvic tilt and gait (antalgic, spastic, wide-based). Look for spinal deformities (scoliosis, gibbus).

Palpation: Gently palpate the entire spine (spinous processes, paraspinal muscles) and sacroiliac areas. Tenderness in the paraspinal muscles or trigger points (e.g. trapezius) suggests strain or myofascial pain. Tenderness at an SI joint (inferior to PSIS) suggests SIJ involvement. Compare active vs passive range of motion: muscle spasm often limits active movement more. In regional exam, the modified Schober's test is typically measured from a point at the lumbosacral junction, with marks 10 cm above and 5 cm below; an increase of less than 5 cm on forward flexion suggests reduced lumbar flexion. Abnormal kyphosis/lordosis should be noted.

Range of motion: Evaluate cervical ROM (flexion, extension, lateral bending, rotation). Spurling's manoeuvre (axial compression with neck extension/rotation) reproducing arm pain indicates cervical radiculopathy. For the thoracic and lumbar spine, measure trunk flexion, extension and lateral bends. Palpate the sacrum/pelvis while the patient moves (Gillet's test: stability of PSIS during hip flexion; restricted motion suggests SIJ dysfunction).

Neurologic exam: Test strength of key myotomes (hip flexors L2–L4, knee extensors L3–L4, dorsiflexors L4–L5, plantar flexors S1, toe extensors L5, hamstrings S2). Check reflexes (patellar L4, Achilles S1). Light touch sensation in dermatomal distributions helps localise nerve root involvement. Upper motor neuron signs (Babinski, clonus, hyperreflexia) indicate spinal cord compression. For cervical pathology, evaluate Hoffmann's sign and coordination.

Special tests: Straight-leg raise and crossed SLR can suggest lumbar nerve root irritation. FABER (flexion-abduction-external rotation) test stresses the SI joint; pain in the SI area is a positive result. Thigh thrust, Gaenslen's test and sacral thrust are other SI provocation manoeuvres; ≥ 3 positive SI tests strongly indicate SIJ pain [4]. Observe chest expansion (measure around T4); a reduced chest expansion (<2 cm) may occur in advanced ankylosing spondylitis. In summary, exam findings often guide further testing, but note that up to 80% of lower back pain cases remain "nonspecific" despite thorough exam.

Role of Imaging and Laboratory Studies

Imaging

Guidelines often recommend against routine imaging in the first 6 weeks of acute low back pain without red flags [7]. Plain radiographs (X-rays) of the spine are indicated if fracture or severe degenerative change is suspected (e.g. after trauma, osteoporosis, chronic steroid use). X-ray can show fractures, advanced osteoarthritis, alignment (spondylolisthesis) and sacroiliitis (graded by modified New York criteria). MRI is the modality of choice when red flags or neurologic deficits are present. MRI visualises discs, ligaments and neural elements; it can detect acute disc herniation, spinal stenosis, infection (discitis/osteomyelitis) and early inflammatory changes (bone marrow oedema in sacroiliitis). CT scan is best for detailed bone anatomy (e.g. fracture assessment) if MRI is contraindicated. Ultrasound is useful for peripheral enthesitis or guidance of injections but has limited role in axial spine diagnosis.

Laboratory

In mechanical/back strains, lab tests are usually normal. However, simple laboratory tests can screen for red flag causes: FBC and inflammatory markers if infection or cancer is a concern. In suspected inflammatory back pain/axial SpA, HLA-B27 testing, CRP and ESR are appropriate. HLA-B27 positivity supports a SpA diagnosis (present in ~90% of AS patients), while a negative result makes it less likely (though not impossible). Elevated CRP or ESR indicates active inflammation but is neither sensitive nor specific (many axial SpA patients have normal ESR/CRP). In suspected infection, CRP/ESR are usually high; blood cultures and specific serologies (e.g. TB) may be needed. For possible malignancy, tests like serum protein electrophoresis (for myeloma), PSA or tumour markers are guided by clinical suspicion. Ultimately, imaging and laboratory tests should be tailored depending on the clinical presentation.

Inflammatory Back Pain/Axial Spondyloarthritis

For chronic back pain, screening for axial SpA is important. Common inflammatory back pain includes insidious onset, morning stiffness, improvement with exercise and nocturnal pain improving on rising.

The ASAS classification criteria can be applied to patients under the age of 45 with over 3 months of back pain. There are a broad range of criteria, but certain features include sacroiliitis on MRI or X-ray, inflammatory back pain, arthritis, enthesitis, anterior uveitis, psoriasis, inflammatory bowel disease, good response to NSAIDs, family history and peripheral arthritis [15]. Other tools like the Bath Ankylosing Spondylitis indices (BASDAI for disease activity, BASFI for function) are used for monitoring, but initial screening focuses on IBP features, HLA-B27 and imaging [16]. Early identification allows treatment before irreversible fusion occurs and therefore better patient outcomes.

Management

Conservative (Non-pharmacologic) Management [17]

Initial management of most spinal pain is conservative. Key principles are patient education and staying active. Patients should be reassured that most back pain improves with time and movement. Advice includes maintaining activity, avoiding bed rest and applying ergonomic measures (proper lifting technique, ergonomic workstations).

Physiotherapy is central: supervised exercise programmes focusing on stretching, core and back strengthening and aerobic conditioning. For example, transversus abdominis and multifidus strengthening (planks, bird-dogs) improve spinal stability, and hamstring/gluteal stretches reduce back strain. Postural training (neutral spine, ergonomic chairs) helps neck and back pain. Cognitive-behavioural therapy or multidisciplinary pain programmes are useful for chronic pain with psychosocial factors. Passive modalities (heat/cold, traction) may provide short-term relief.

In general, active rehabilitation (exercise therapy, physiotherapy) has the best evidence in chronic lower back pain. Patient education about the benign nature of most back pain and realistic prognosis is essential.

Manual Therapy and Trigger Point Injections

Manual therapies can be adjuncts. Options include spinal manipulation or mobilisation, massage, acupuncture and osteopathic techniques. The evidence is mixed: for some patients, manipulation may reduce acute pain, but benefits are modest and short term [18]. Massage and myofascial release can relieve muscle tension in the trapezius, paraspinals or gluteals. Occupational therapy may address workplace ergonomics.

For myofascial trigger points, conservative measures are first line: stretching, posture correction, physiotherapy and relaxation. If severe, injections of local anaesthetic (with or without steroid) into trigger points can be considered, but evidence is limited. Trigger-point injections yield modest, short-term pain reduction and should be reserved for refractory cases [19]. No medication (lidocaine, steroids, dry needling) has proven superior.

For suspected SIJ or facet joint pain, diagnostic blocks could be considered. Intraarticular SIJ steroid injections under fluoroscopic guidance can confirm SIJ as pain source and provide relief. Chronic SIJ pain may be treated with cooled radio-frequency ablation (RFA) of lateral branch nerves pain is sometimes diagnosed by medial branch blocks; a positive test followed by medial branch RFA can yield relief. In summary, interventions like injections and RFA are options for refractory pain after conservative treatment fails, but they are selected case by case.

Pharmacological Management [20]

Medications are adjuncts for pain control. *NSAIDs* are often used first line for both mechanical and inflammatory pain because of their analgesic and anti-inflammatory effects.

Analgesics: Paracetamol has little evidence in back pain. Opioids provide short-term relief in severe acute pain but carry risk; they are not recommended for chronic lower back pain management. Muscle relaxants (e.g. cyclobenzaprine, tizanidine) may help acute muscle spasm, but evidence is weak and sedation common. Antidepressants or anticonvulsants are not routinely indicated unless for neuropathic pain.

Steroids: Systemic steroids are generally ineffective for chronic low back pain. A short course of oral steroids is sometimes used for severe inflammatory flares. Epidural steroid injections may be tried for radicular pain (with mixed evidence), and facet joint steroid injections can be diagnostic/therapeutic.

If axial SpA is confirmed, treatment escalates. Conventional DMARDs (methotrexate, sulfasalazine) are not effective for axial disease, though sulfasalazine may help peripheral arthritis. The mainstay in active axial SpA (refractory to NSAIDs) is biologic therapy. Tumour necrosis factor (TNF) inhibitors (etanercept, adalimumab, infliximab, certolizumab, golimumab) are highly effective for axial symptoms and extraspinal manifestations. UK treatment pathways recommend biologic or targeted synthetic therapy for active axial SpA when disease remains active despite adequate NSAID trials, under specialist supervision [21]. Newer interleukin-17 inhibitors (secukinumab, ixekizumab) are also approved for axial SpA [22]. These agents require specialist prescription.

Indications for Referral

Referral pathways depend on urgency and aetiology.

Urgent referral: Any red flag finding (cauda equina, myelopathy, suspected infection or fracture) warrants immediate emergency or spine surgery evaluation.

Rheumatology referral: Patients with chronic inflammatory back pain features (especially age <45, HLA-B27+, elevated CRP) should be referred to a rheumatologist for axial SpA workup.

Pain/surgery referral: Most mechanical lower back pain is managed nonsurgically. Surgery is rarely indicated, typically for intractable pain after >1 year or progressive neurologic deficit. Multidisciplinary pain management programmes (physiatry/pain clinics) can be beneficial for chronic disabling pain. If conservative measures (PT, medications) fail to control severe pain, referral to orthopaedics or pain specialists (for advanced imaging, injections or consideration of fusion/RFA) may be appropriate.

Rehabilitation and Prognosis

Rehabilitation for chronic axial pain is multidisciplinary. Emphasise long-term exercise therapy, patient education and psychosocial support. Cardiovascular fitness (walking, swimming) and core stabilisation exercises (planks, bridges) improve outcomes. Weight loss and smoking cessation enhance recovery. Cognitive-behavioural therapy and pain-coping programmes are useful when pain becomes chronic and disabling.

Prognosis varies by cause. Acute mechanical back pain often improves: about 90% of patients recover within 6 weeks [23]. However, recurrence is common, with roughly 24–80% experiencing another episode within a year [24]. Most residual disability is low with proper rehab. Axial SpA, on the other hand, is chronic and may gradually progress. Early and appropriate therapy (NSAIDs, biologics, exercise) can dramatically reduce symptoms and maintain function, but some patients develop permanent changes (vertebral fusion). With modern biologic treatments, many patients achieve good symptom control or remission. Ongoing management includes monitoring for complications (osteoporosis, cardiovascular risk) and encouraging spinal mobility (e.g. chest expansion exercises). Overall, patient education about realistic goals and self-management is key in rehabilitation.

Key Learning Points

- The spine's normal curves (cervical/lumbar lordosis, thoracic kyphosis) and segmental anatomy (vertebrae, discs, facets) determine motion and load distribution. Paraspinal muscles (erector spinae, multifidus) and core muscles provide dynamic stability.
- *Soft tissue pain*: Muscle strains and myofascial trigger points in cervical or lumbar paraspinals (e.g. trapezius, quadratus lumborum, thoracolumbar fascia) are common sources of neck/back pain. Sacroiliac joint dysfunction also mimics mechanical lower back pain.

- *Mechanical* vs *inflammatory*: Mechanical back pain is typically acute and activity-related, improves with rest and has normal laboratory tests. Inflammatory back pain (axSpA) is insidious, age <40, lasts >3 months, with morning stiffness and improvement with exercise. HLA-B27 positivity and elevated CRP/ESR (when present) support inflammatory causes.
- *Red flags*: Progressive neurologic deficits (e.g. cauda equina), systemic symptoms (fever, weight loss), history of cancer, IV drug use and severe trauma warrant urgent evaluation (imaging, referral).
- *Exam*: Perform a thorough spine exam with ROM, palpation of muscles/spine and neurologic testing. Special tests include Spurling's (cervical radiculopathy), straight-leg raise (lumbar radiculopathy) and SIJ provocation (FABER, Gaenslen).
- *Imaging*: Reserve imaging for red flags or persistent pain (>6–12 weeks). X-rays detect fractures, severe arthritis or gross sacroiliitis. MRI is best for neural or soft tissue pathology (disc herniation, infection, early sacroiliitis). Ultrasound can image peripheral enthesitis but has limited axial role.
- *Laboratory tests*: Consider HLA-B27 and inflammatory markers if axial SpA is suspected. Note that CRP/ESR may be normal even in active disease. CBC, calcium, PSA or SPEP are used if malignancy/infection is suspected.
- *Management*: Emphasise conservative therapy. Regular exercise, posture correction and core strengthening are mainstays. Manual therapies/massage can relieve muscle pain. Pharmacologically, NSAIDs are first line (effective in both mechanical pain and AS). Analgesics and muscle relaxants have limited evidence. Biologics (TNF or IL-17 inhibitors) are indicated for axial SpA unresponsive to NSAIDs.
- *Referral*: Urgent referral for red flag cases. Refer to rheumatology if inflammatory back pain is likely (positive ASAS criteria, HLA-B27). Chronic disabling pain unresponsive to conservative care may merit specialist evaluation.
- *Prognosis*: Most acute lower back pain resolves with conservative care; chronic pain can recur. Axial SpA is a lifelong condition; with treatment, many patients achieve good function, but some limitations may remain.

References

1. Rahman S, Das JM. Anatomy, head and neck: cervical spine [Internet]. In: StatPearls; 2026. Available from: http://www.ncbi.nlm.nih.gov/pubmed/21508286.
2. Waxenbaum JA, Reddy V, Margetis K. Anatomy, back, thoracic vertebrae [Internet]. In: StatPearls; 2026. Available from: http://www.ncbi.nlm.nih.gov/pubmed/29959309.
3. Hashmi SS, Seifert KD, Massoud TF. Thoracic and lumbosacral spine anatomy. Neuroimaging Clin N Am [Internet]. 2022;32(4):889–902. Available from: http://www.ncbi.nlm.nih.gov/pubmed/36244729
4. Forst SL, Wheeler MT, Fortin JD, Vilensky JA. The sacroiliac joint: anatomy, physiology and clinical significance. Pain Physician [Internet]. 2006;9(1):61–7. Available from: http://www.ncbi.nlm.nih.gov/pubmed/16700283
5. Jaumard NV, Welch WC, Winkelstein BA. Spinal facet joint biomechanics and mechanotransduction in normal, injury and degenerative conditions. J Biomech Eng [Internet]. 2011;133(7):071010. Available from: http://www.ncbi.nlm.nih.gov/pubmed/21823749

6. Henson B, Kadiyala B, Edens MA. Anatomy, back, muscles [internet]. In: StatPearls; 2026. Available from: http://www.ncbi.nlm.nih.gov/pubmed/33038198.
7. Will JS, Bury DC, Miller JA. Mechanical low back pain. Am Fam Physician [Internet]. 2018;98(7):421–8. Available from: http://www.ncbi.nlm.nih.gov/pubmed/30252425
8. Raj MA, Ampat G, Varacallo MA. Sacroiliac joint pain [Internet]. In: StatPearls; 2026. Available from: http://www.ncbi.nlm.nih.gov/pubmed/16244008.
9. Saueressig T, Owen PJ, Diemer F, Zebisch J, Belavy DL. Diagnostic accuracy of clusters of pain provocation tests for detecting sacroiliac joint pain: systematic review with meta-analysis. J Orthop Sports Phys Ther [Internet]. 2021;51(9):422–31. Available from: http://www.ncbi.nlm.nih.gov/pubmed/34210160
10. Navarro-Compán V, Sepriano A, El-Zorkany B, van der Heijde D. Axial spondyloarthritis. Ann Rheum Dis [Internet]. 2021;80(12):1511–21. Available from: http://www.ncbi.nlm.nih.gov/pubmed/34615639
11. Biggioggero M, Crotti C, Becciolini A, Miserocchi E, Favalli EG. The management of acute anterior uveitis complicating Spondyloarthritis: present and future. Biomed Res Int [Internet]. 2018;2018:9460187. Available from: http://www.ncbi.nlm.nih.gov/pubmed/30406148
12. Sieper J, Braun J, Rudwaleit M, Boonen A, Zink A. Ankylosing spondylitis: an overview. Ann Rheum Dis [Internet]. 2002;61 Suppl 3:iii8–18. Available from: http://www.ncbi.nlm.nih.gov/pubmed/12381506
13. Lorenzin M, Ometto F, Ortolan A, Felicetti M, Favero M, Doria A, et al. An update on serum biomarkers to assess axial spondyloarthritis and to guide treatment decision. Ther Adv Musculoskelet Dis [Internet]. 2020;12:1759720X20934277. Available from: http://www.ncbi.nlm.nih.gov/pubmed/32636944
14. Rudwaleit M, van der Heijde D, Landewe R, Listing J, Akkoc N, Brandt J, et al. The development of Assessment of SpondyloArthritis international Society classification criteria for axial spondyloarthritis (part II): validation and final selection. Ann Rheum Dis [Internet]. 2009;68(6):777–83. Available from: http://ard.bmj.com/cgi/doi/10.1136/ard.2009.108233
15. Sieper J, Rudwaleit M, Baraliakos X, Brandt J, Braun J, Burgos-Vargas R, et al. The Assessment of SpondyloArthritis international Society (ASAS) handbook: a guide to assess spondyloarthritis. Ann Rheum Dis [Internet]. 2009;68 Suppl 2:ii1–44. Available from: http://www.ncbi.nlm.nih.gov/pubmed/19433414
16. Garrett S, Jenkinson T, Kennedy LG, Whitelock H, Gaisford P, Calin A. A new approach to defining disease status in ankylosing spondylitis: the Bath Ankylosing Spondylitis Disease Activity Index. J Rheumatol [Internet]. 1994;21(12):2286–91. Available from: http://www.ncbi.nlm.nih.gov/pubmed/7699630
17. Lee SW, Nguyen D, Mack D, Aguila E, Thomas M, Doddy K. Conservative management of low back pain. HCA Healthc J Med [Internet]. 2021;2(5):319–28. Available from: http://www.ncbi.nlm.nih.gov/pubmed/37425131
18. Grenier J-P, Rothmund M. A critical review of the role of manual therapy in the treatment of individuals with low back pain. J Man Manip Ther [Internet]. 2024;32(5):464–77. Available from: http://www.ncbi.nlm.nih.gov/pubmed/38381584
19. Hammi C, Schroeder JD, Yeung B. Trigger point injection [Internet]. In: StatPearls; 2026. Available from: http://www.ncbi.nlm.nih.gov/pubmed/17321283.
20. Cashin AG, Wand BM, O'Connell NE, Lee H, Rizzo RR, Bagg MK, et al. Pharmacological treatments for low back pain in adults: an overview of Cochrane reviews. Cochrane Database Syst Rev [Internet]. 2023;4(4):CD013815. Available from: http://www.ncbi.nlm.nih.gov/pubmed/37014979
21. National Institute For Health and Care Excellence. TNF-alpha inhibitors for ankylosing spondylitis and non-radiographic axial spondyloarthritis. NICE Guid [Internet]; 2016. Available from: https://www.nice.org.uk/guidance/ta383/chapter/1-Recommendations
22. National Institute For Health and Care Excellence. Secukinumab for active ankylosing spondylitis after treatment with non-steroidal anti-inflammatory drugs or TNF-alpha inhibitors [Internet]; 2019. Available from: https://www.nice.org.uk/guidance/ta407/chapter/1-Recommendations

23. da C Menezes Costa L, Maher CG, Hancock MJ, JH MA, Herbert RD, Costa LOP. The prognosis of acute and persistent low-back pain: a meta-analysis. CMAJ [Internet]. 2012;184(11):E613–24. Available from: http://www.ncbi.nlm.nih.gov/pubmed/22586331
24. Hoy D, Brooks P, Blyth F, Buchbinder R. The epidemiology of low back pain. Best Pract Res Clin Rheumatol [Internet]. 2010;24(6):769–81. Available from: http://www.ncbi.nlm.nih.gov/pubmed/21665125

Hip and Pelvic Girdle Soft Tissue Syndromes

8

Abstract

Hip and pelvic girdle soft tissue syndromes are common causes of lateral and buttock pain in adults, especially middle-aged women and older adults. These conditions include greater trochanteric pain syndrome (GTPS, encompassing gluteal medius/minimus tendinopathy and trochanteric bursitis), iliopsoas tendinopathy, piriformis syndrome and proximal hamstring tendinopathy. This chapter reviews their anatomy, biomechanics, clinical presentation, diagnosis and management. Key differences from hip joint pathology (e.g. osteoarthritis, labral tears) and spinal disorders (e.g. lumbar radiculopathy, stenosis) are highlighted. History and focused physical exam manoeuvres—such as palpation of the greater trochanter, resistance tests for hip abduction/flexion and special tests like the FABER and FAIR manoeuvres—can help pinpoint the source of pain (Pumarejo Gomez L et al., Greater trochanteric pain syndrome (Greater trochanteric bursitis). StatPearls, 2026; Sunil Kumar KH et al., Knee Surg Sports Traumatol Arthrosc 29(8):2408–2416, 2021). Diagnostic imaging is mainly used to confirm or exclude pathology: ultrasound and MRI can reveal gluteal or hamstring tendon tears and bursitis, whereas X-rays assess joint arthritis or bony impingement (Chamberlain R, Am Fam Physician 103(2):81–89, 2021). Initial management is usually conservative (physiotherapy with targeted strengthening and stretching, NSAIDs, activity modification); image-guided injections (e.g. trochanteric bursa or piriformis injection) provide symptom relief in many cases. Surgical referral is reserved for rare refractory cases (e.g. endoscopic gluteal tendon repair). Prognosis is generally good with proper therapy, and prevention focuses on addressing contributing factors like muscle imbalances, biomechanics and overuse. This chapter provides a comprehensive, clinically focused overview of hip and pelvic soft tissue syndromes, integrating anatomy with evidence-based diagnosis and treatment strategies (Reid D, J Orthop 13(1):15–28, 2016).

© The Author(s), under exclusive license to Springer Nature Switzerland AG 2026

R. Amarnani, *Soft Tissue and Musculoskeletal Medicine in Rheumatology*,
https://doi.org/10.1007/978-3-032-29441-8_8

Clinical Vignette

Mrs. B is a 68-year-old woman who presents with a 6-month history of progressive right hip pain. The pain is described as a deep ache over the outside of her right hip, worse when lying on that side at night or climbing stairs and sometimes radiating to the mid-thigh. She denies any trauma. Her past history is notable for mild knee osteoarthritis. On examination, there is focal tenderness over the right greater trochanter. Passive hip flexion, adduction and internal rotation are not limited (negative FADIR test), but resisted hip abduction reproduces her lateral hip pain. She has a positive FABER (flexion-abduction-external rotation) test on the right, provoking similar discomfort. Trendelenburg test (single-leg stand) is normal. Strength of hip abduction is only slightly reduced due to pain. Gait is mildly antalgic on the right. There is no back pain or neurologic deficits.

Given the history and exam, greater trochanteric pain syndrome is suspected rather than hip arthritis or lumbar radiculopathy [1]. The patient is advised on activity modification and starts a course of targeted physiotherapy focusing on gluteal strengthening. She is given an NSAID for pain. Over the next several weeks, her pain improves but does not fully resolve. A diagnostic ultrasound is obtained, showing tendinosis of the gluteus medius tendon with subgluteus medius bursal fluid. Ultrasound-guided corticosteroid injection into the trochanteric bursa is performed, leading to significant pain relief. Over months she gradually returns to normal activity. This case illustrates the typical clinical features, differential diagnosis and treatment pathway for lateral hip soft tissue pain in an older adult.

Anatomy and Biomechanics of the Hip and Pelvic Girdle

The hip and pelvic girdle comprise the bony pelvis (ilium, ischium, pubis and sacrum), the hip joints and multiple musculotendinous structures that stabilise and move the lower limb [2]. The hip joint is a ball-and-socket joint between the femoral head and the acetabulum of the pelvis, allowing flexion/extension, abduction/adduction and internal/external rotation. Surrounding this joint are several muscles and tendons relevant to soft tissue syndromes:

- *Gluteal tendons and bursae* (Fig. 8.1): The gluteus medius and minimus muscles arise from the lateral ilium and insert onto the greater trochanter of the femur, providing hip abduction and pelvic stabilisation during gait [3, 4]. The gluteus maximus originates from the posterior ilium and sacrum and inserts into the iliotibial band (ITB) and gluteal tuberosity of femur, contributing to hip extension and external rotation. The iliotibial band runs down the lateral thigh, thickening over the greater trochanter. Over these tendon insertions lie the greater trochanteric and subgluteus medius bursae, which reduce friction. GTPS (greater trochanteric pain syndrome) (trochanteric bursitis/gluteal tendinopathy) involves pathology of these tendons or bursae [5] (Fig. 8.1).

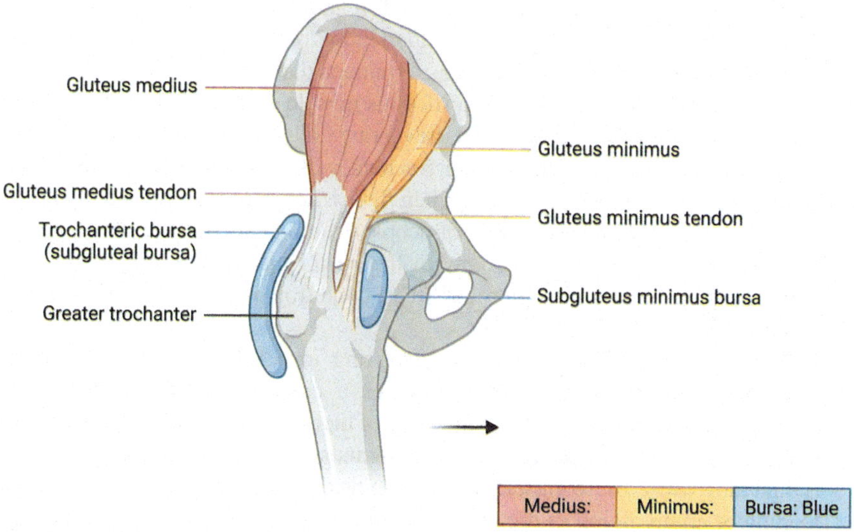

Fig. 8.1 Anatomy of the gluteal tendons (gluteus medius/minimus) and the greater trochanteric bursa

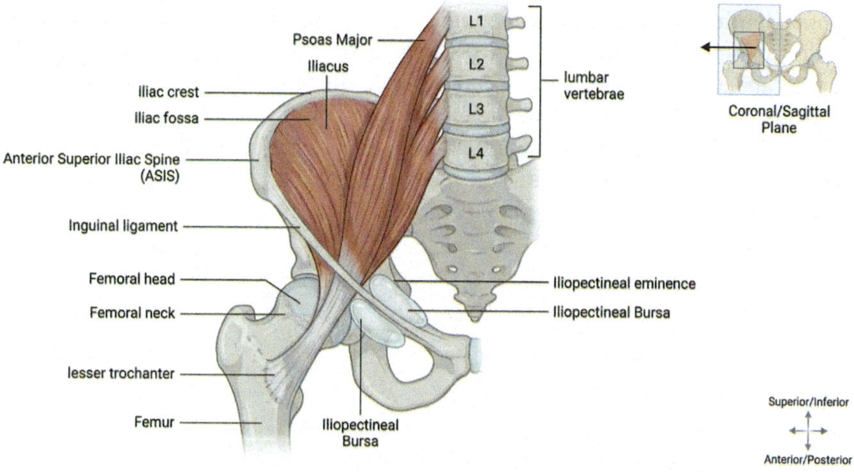

Fig. 8.2 Anatomy of the iliopsoas muscle, tendon and iliopectineal bursa

- *Iliopsoas tendon and bursa* (Fig. 8.2): The iliopsoas muscle is the primary hip flexor. It consists of the iliacus (from the iliac fossa) and psoas major (from lumbar vertebrae), which converge to insert on the lesser trochanter of the femur [6]. Just anterior to the hip joint, the iliopsoas tendon slides over the iliopectineal eminence; a bursa separates it from the joint capsule. Iliopsoas tendinopathy or bursitis (often called "iliopsoas syndrome") presents as anterior groin pain [7].

Biomechanically, the iliopsoas flexes the hip and assists in maintaining lumbar lordosis. Overuse or impingement of the tendon/bursa can occur with repeated hip extension or forceful flexion (e.g. in runners, dancers).

- *Piriformis and sciatic nerve*: The piriformis muscle originates from the anterior sacrum and sacrotuberous ligament, traversing the greater sciatic notch to insert on the superior aspect of the greater trochanter [8]. It externally rotates the hip when extended and abducts the hip when flexed. The sciatic nerve usually passes inferior to the piriformis (in ~80% of people), running deep in the gluteal region (Fig. 8.3). Tightness or hypertrophy of the piriformis can compress the sciatic nerve, causing "piriformis syndrome". This condition often mimics sciatica from a lumbar source.
- *Hamstring tendons* (Fig. 8.3): The hamstring muscle group (biceps femoris, semitendinosus, semimembranosus) shares a common origin on the ischial tuberosity of the pelvis [9]. The long head of biceps femoris and semitendinosus attach to the lateral facet and semimembranosus to the medial aspect of the ischial tuberosity. These muscles act in knee flexion and hip extension. Repetitive loading or compression of the proximal hamstring tendons (e.g. during running or prolonged sitting) can lead to "high hamstring (ischial) tendinopathy". Their poor blood supply at the origin predisposes them to degenerative tendinopathy.

Biomechanics During gait and single-leg stance, the hip abductors (gluteus medius/minimus) counter the pelvis dropping on the contralateral side. Weak or injured abductors lead to compensatory pelvic tilt (Trendelenburg gait) [10]. The iliopsoas is critical for lifting the leg forward. The piriformis contributes to stabilising the femoral head within the acetabulum and controls external rotation; it can become overactive or tight with hip muscle imbalance. Hamstrings eccentrically

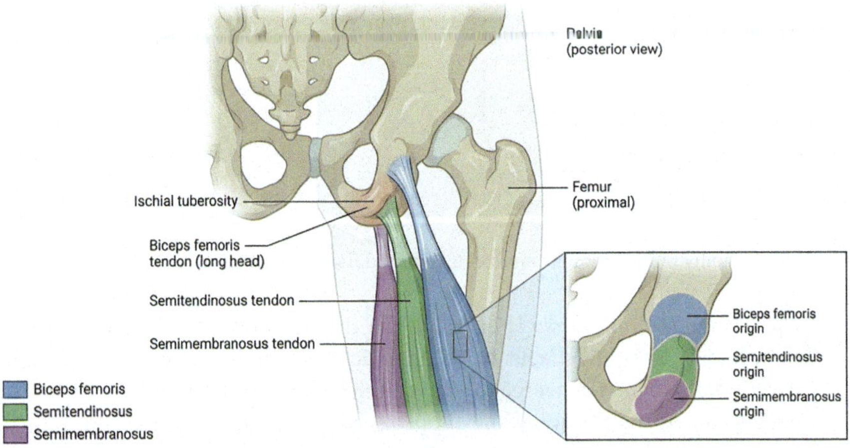

Fig. 8.3 Origin of the hamstring tendons (biceps femoris, semitendinosus, semimembranosus) at the ischial tuberosity

decelerate knee extension in swing phase. Imbalances or overuse of any of these muscles, as well as altered biomechanics (leg length discrepancy, pelvic obliquity), can increase stress on tendons and bursae, predisposing to tendinopathy or bursitis [2]. Women may be at higher risk because of differences in pelvic morphology, hip biomechanics and compressive loading across the gluteal tendons [11]. Overall, understanding these anatomy and function relationships is crucial for diagnosing and treating soft tissue hip syndromes.

Common Soft Tissue Syndromes

Greater Trochanteric Pain Syndrome (GTPS): Gluteal Tendinopathy and Trochanteric Bursitis

Definition and Epidemiology GTPS is an umbrella term for pathology of the hip abductor region, most commonly gluteus medius/minimus tendinopathy or tear, with or without trochanteric bursitis. It is a common source of lateral hip pain, affecting about 15% of women and 8% of men [3]. The classic patient is a middle-aged or older woman with insidious onset of lateral hip pain. Risk factors include female sex, high BMI, iliotibial band tightness, gluteal weakness and hip osteoarthritis or femoroacetabular impingement as contributing factors.

Pathophysiology Contrary to its former name ("trochanteric bursitis"), imaging studies show that primary bursitis is uncommon. In a large series of GTPS patients, only ~20% had evidence of trochanteric bursal inflammation; by contrast, nearly 50% had gluteal tendinosis and 28% had a thickened iliotibial band [12]. Thus, GTPS usually stems from chronic overload and degeneration (tendinopathy) of the gluteus medius/minimus tendons at their trochanteric insertions, often accompanied by secondary bursal fluid from friction [3]. Gluteal tendon tears (partial or full-thickness) occur, especially in the anterior fibres of the medius, and resemble a "rotator cuff tear of the hip." Anatomical factors like a thickened IT band or pelvic tilt can further compress the tendons. Microtrauma triggers a cycle of tendon degeneration: collagen disorganisation, increased type III collagen, neovascularisation and hypercellularity, without a robust inflammatory response [13]. In practice, many patients have gluteal tendinopathy (with or without minor tears) leading to chronic lateral hip pain, with bursitis as a secondary finding in a minority.

Clinical Presentation [14] GTPS typically causes a burning or aching pain localised to the lateral hip (greater trochanter) that can radiate down the lateral thigh and occasionally into the buttock or knee. Pain worsens with lying on the affected side, prolonged standing, stair climbing or any activity requiring hip abduction. Patients often report difficulty sleeping on the painful hip. On exam, there is point tenderness directly over the greater trochanter. Palpation may evoke a "jump sign" (patient involuntarily raises away). Resisted hip abduction or external rotation against resistance usually reproduces the pain. Hip abductor weakness may be present; severe cases show a Trendelenburg gait or positive single-leg-stance test. The FABER (Patrick) test is often positive in GTPS, whereas internal hip rotation pain is more characteristic of joint pathology. Other common findings include tightness of the iliotibial band (positive Ober's test) and pain with resisted external derotation of the hip. Importantly, GTPS must be distinguished from other causes of lateral hip pain. In contrast to hip osteoarthritis (groin/internal rotation pain, morning stiffness) or lumbar radiculopathy (leg pain below knee, neurologic symptoms), GTPS pain is specifically localised to the trochanteric region and worsened by direct compression or use of the abductors.

Imaging Imaging for GTPS is guided by clinical suspicion. Ultrasound can detect tendinopathic changes (tendon thickening, hypoechogenicity) or tears in the gluteus medius/minimus, as well as trochanteric bursal fluid. An MRI of the hip is more sensitive for partial or full-thickness gluteal tears, abductor muscle atrophy and bursitis. For example, ultrasound/MRI will often show no bursitis in the majority of GTPS cases [12]. X-rays are usually unremarkable for soft tissue causes but are indicated to assess for hip osteoarthritis, femoroacetabular impingement (e.g. cam/pincer lesions) or avascular necrosis, which can present similarly. In practice, if GTPS is strongly suspected clinically, a diagnostic ultrasound or MRI is obtained only if the diagnosis is unclear or surgery is being considered.

Management Initial treatment is conservative. Load management (reducing aggravating activities), NSAIDs or paracetamol for pain and ice can be helpful. A structured physiotherapy programme is central to recovery: it emphasises hip abductor and core strengthening and eccentric loading of the gluteal tendons. Avoid positions that excessively compress the gluteal tendons, such as prolonged hip adduction or lying directly on the affected side. Flexibility work should be gentle and symptom-guided rather than aggressive ITB stretching. Strengthening the gluteus medius (e.g. side-lying hip raises, resisted bands) and balance exercises correct the underlying abductor weakness. Low-energy extracorporeal shock wave therapy (ESWT) has shown benefit in some studies as an adjunct for refractory GTPS.

If pain persists, image-guided injections may be used. Steroid (plus anaesthetic) injection into the greater trochanteric bursa provides short-term relief, especially if bursitis is present. However, studies suggest superior long-term improvement when treating tendon pathology directly (e.g. peritendinous injection around the gluteus medius tendon) rather than the superficial bursa [15]. For persistent gluteal tendinopathy, some clinicians use ultrasound-guided platelet-rich plasma (PRP) or percutaneous needle fenestration of the tendon (tenotomy) techniques [16]. Injections for bursitis/tendinopathy can usually be done under ultrasound guidance for accuracy. Surgical referral is considered in rare refractory cases: endoscopic (arthroscopic) trochanteric bursectomy and gluteus medius repair has been successful in severe tears [17].

Iliopsoas (Anterior Hip) Tendinopathy

Definition and Pathology Iliopsoas tendinopathy (iliopsoas bursitis/syndrome) is an uncommon but important cause of anterior (groin) hip pain. It often coexists with snapping hip (the iliopsoas tendon snapping over the iliopectineal eminence) and has been termed "iliopsoas syndrome" [18]. Causes include overuse (e.g. running, ballet, kicking sports), hip flexor tightness and prior hip surgery. Pathologically, the iliopsoas tendon or its bursa becomes irritated, leading to pain and occasionally localised inflammation. Unlike GTPS, iliopsoas issues are less about degeneration and more about mechanical overload or impingement of the tendon.

Clinical Features [19] Patients with iliopsoas tendinopathy report deep groin or anterior hip pain, exacerbated by hip flexion activities (e.g. climbing stairs, sitting up, getting in/out of a car). Some describe a snapping or catching sensation in the front of the hip. On exam, there may be tenderness along the iliopsoas tendon (just distal to the inguinal crease or in the groin region). The Thomas test (pain on extending the hip from a supine flexion position) may be positive due to psoas irritation. Resisted hip flexion (especially at 90° flexion) often reproduces pain. Unlike hip joint pathology, there is usually no limitation of hip internal rotation. Sometimes the pain can refer to the anteromedial thigh. Because iliopsoas pain is deep, many cases are initially misdiagnosed as hip joint pain or even femoroacetabular impingement. However, the lack of radiographic joint changes and a normal internal rotation range help differentiate it. Imaging is primarily diagnostic: ultrasound can show fluid in the iliopsoas bursa or thickened tendon, and MRI (or MR arthrography) may show inflammation of the tendon or bursa. MRI/CT have limited roles except to rule out other pathology [20].

Management Conservative therapy is first line [18]. This includes iliopsoas stretching exercises (hip extension stretches), core and hip flexor strengthening and anti-inflammatory medications. Activity modification (avoiding hip hyperextension) is advised. Image-guided corticosteroid injection into the iliopsoas bursa (via ultrasound or fluoroscopy) can provide significant relief in stubborn cases [21]; success rates for guided iliopsoas injections are high, especially in patients with hip arthroplasty-related tendinitis [22]. If conservative measures fail and symptoms are disabling, surgical release of the iliopsoas tendon (via open or arthroscopic approach) can be considered, though outcomes are variable. In practice, most patients improve gradually with physiotherapy and targeted injections.

Proximal Hamstring (Ischial) Tendinopathy

Definition and Pathology Proximal hamstring tendinopathy (sometimes called high hamstring or hamstring origin tendinopathy) involves chronic degeneration at the origin of the hamstring muscles on the ischial tuberosity [9]. It often occurs in athletes (runners, sprinters, hockey, soccer) with repetitive hip flexion and knee extension but can also affect sedentary people. Compression of the hamstring tendons against the pelvis during hip flexion is thought to initiate pathology [23]. Over time, the tendon develops collagen degeneration, neovascularisation and even partial tearing near its attachment. A related neuropathy ("proximal hamstring tendinopathy-related sciatic nerve entrapment") can arise from fibrotic tissue between the semimembranosus tendon and the sciatic nerve.

Clinical Presentation Patients report a deep, aching buttock or upper posterior thigh pain centred over the ischial tuberosity [24]. Pain is aggravated by activities such as running, lunging, squatting and especially prolonged sitting (sitting increases compression of the ischial area). On exam, palpation of the ischial tuberosity reproduces pain. Passive straight leg raise may be limited by pain or tightness, and hamstring stretching (forward trunk bend or bent-knee stretch test) elicits discomfort. Resisted knee flexion in prone can cause pain at the ischial origin. Unlike hamstring muscle strains, there is usually no acute "pop" history; pain is insidious. Hip range of motion is full, and there are no true neurological deficits. Imaging by MRI or ultrasound often shows thickening and increased signal in the proximal hamstring tendons, with possible partial tears or bursitis (ischial bursitis may coexist).

Management Treatment is primarily nonoperative [25]. Rehabilitation focuses on eccentric loading of the hamstrings, hip extensor strengthening and lumbopelvic stabilisation exercises to offload the tendon attachment. Phased rehab programs (progressing from isometrics to isotonic to energy-storage loading) have been described. Stretching exercises for the hamstrings and gluteal muscles are incorporated carefully to avoid overlengthening the tendon. Activity modification (reducing running/well bending) is advised. NSAIDs and ice can control pain during acute flares.

If persistent, image-guided corticosteroid injection at the ischial tuberosity (into the tendon sheath/bursa) may relieve symptoms. The literature on injection efficacy is mixed; one study showed that some patients get short-term relief from steroid injection [25]. Platelet-rich plasma and shockwave therapy are sometimes used, though evidence is limited. Overall, most patients improve over months with structured rehab; return to sport is usually possible with adequate strengthening. Persistence or recurrence of symptoms is not uncommon if underlying mechanics are not corrected.

Differentiating Soft Tissue Conditions from Hip Joint Pathology and Spinal Pain

A thorough differential diagnosis is essential for hip and pelvic soft tissue pain. Key features help distinguish these from intraarticular hip disease and referred pain:

- *Hip joint pathology (e.g. osteoarthritis, labral tear, FAI)*: These typically present with groin or anterior thigh pain rather than isolated lateral pain [14]. There is often morning stiffness, limited internal rotation and positive impingement tests (FADIR provokes groin pain). Patients may report locking or clicking (labral tear) or difficulty with pivoting movements (FAI). Importantly, a common question is ability to put on shoes/socks: inability suggests hip joint involvement. Imaging (X-ray or MRI) will show joint space narrowing or labral injury. In contrast, GTPS patients can usually don socks without groin pain and have minimal limitation of hip range [3].
- *Lumbar spine referral*: Pain from lumbar radiculopathy or spinal stenosis often radiates below the knee and is associated with back pain, numbness or tingling and is worse with spine extension or certain postures [8]. Neurological examination may reveal sensory or reflex changes in a dermatomal pattern. Hip vs spine differentiation hinges on pain location and aggravating factors: true sciatic pain involves foot or calf tingling, whereas lateral hip soft tissue pain rarely extends past the knee. Tests like straight-leg raise (SLR) and spinal exam help; a normal spine exam with lateral hip tenderness points away from discogenic pain.
- *Sacroiliac (SI) joint dysfunction* [26]: SI pain can cause buttock/hip pain but tends to be slightly more posterior and can be reproduced by SI provocation tests (e.g. FABER, Gaenslen). There may be concomitant low back pain.
- *Other soft tissue*: IT band syndrome causes lateral knee pain rather than hip pain. Hip flexor strains may present with groin pain (not lateral). Greater trochanteric bursitis, vs iliopsoas, vs piriformis, etc. is determined by specific exam. For example, active resisted hip abduction elicits GTPS pain, whereas resisted flexion targets iliopsoas or rectus femoris.

In summary, careful history of pain location, severity (aggravating activities like lying on the side vs sitting), and focused exam manoeuvres (FABER, FADIR, Trendelenburg, SLR, palpation points) can usually differentiate soft tissue hip syndromes from joint or spine aetiologies. Imaging then confirms the suspected diagnosis or rules out mimic conditions.

History and Physical Examination

A structured history and physical exam are vital for diagnosing hip/pelvic soft tissue syndromes. Key historical points include duration and onset of pain, aggravating activities (e.g. weight-bearing, sitting, lying on hip, sports) and any injury. For each syndrome, note specific features: for example, lateral hip pain on side-lying suggests GTPS; anterior groin pain with hip flexion suggests iliopsoas; buttock pain with sitting suggests piriformis; deep posterior thigh pain after running or with sitting suggests hamstring origin. Inquire about systemic symptoms (fever, systemic arthritis) and spine or knee issues.

Physical examination should start with observation of gait and posture. Look for Trendelenburg gait (pelvic drop on contralateral side) indicating abductor weakness. Assess leg lengths and pelvic tilt. Examine the lumbar spine and SI joints to exclude spine referral. Palpate key landmarks: the greater trochanter (tender in GTPS), the groin and lesser trochanter area (iliopsoas), the ischial tuberosity (hamstrings), the sciatic notch/buttock (piriformis) and the SI joint.

Perform resisted muscle tests: hip abduction against resistance aggravates gluteal tendinopathy; resisted hip flexion (especially at 90°) tests iliopsoas; resisted knee flexion checks hamstrings. Range of motion tests: internal rotation of the hip provokes arthritis; FADIR (flexion-adduction-internal rotation) can reproduce FAI or iliopsoas pain (if pain anterior); FABER (flexion-abduction-external rotation) stresses the trochanteric bursa and SI joint. A positive Ober test (unable to adduct knee) suggests IT band tightness often seen with gluteal overload [27]. The bent-knee stretch test (Hamstring stretch test) may reproduce proximal hamstring pain. Documenting muscle strength is important: gluteus medius weakness (or Trendelenburg sign) may indicate a full-thickness tear of that tendon [10].

Neurological exam should be normal in isolated soft tissue syndromes. Check dermatomes and reflexes to rule out radiculopathy. If sensory deficits are present, consider spine or more proximal nerve compression.

In summary, the exam should systematically reproduce or alleviate symptoms with specific manoeuvres: tenderness at the painful site (trochanter, groin, ischium), pain with resisted movements of the implicated muscle and special tests that increase tension on the suspect structure. The constellation of these findings pinpoints the diagnosis.

Imaging Findings

Ultrasound High-resolution ultrasound is excellent for real-time evaluation of tendons and bursae around the hip. It can identify gluteus medius/minimus tendinosis or tears (with hypoechoic or disrupted fibres) and detect trochanteric or iliopsoas bursitis (fluid collection). It also guides injections. For instance, ultrasound has shown that many patients with lateral hip pain have gluteal tendon pathology even when bursitis is minimal [12]. Ultrasound is user-dependent but has the advantage of comparing to the asymptomatic side and performing dynamic assessment (e.g. snapping of iliopsoas).

Magnetic Resonance Imaging (MRI) MRI provides a comprehensive view of soft tissues. In GTPS, MRI can confirm gluteal tendon tears, tendinosis (increased signal on T2-weighted images) and bursal fluid. It can also reveal fatty atrophy of the gluteal muscles in chronic cases. In iliopsoas syndromes, MRI may show thickened tendon or increased bursal fluid between iliopsoas and the joint. For piriformis syndrome, advanced MRI neurography may demonstrate nerve swelling or signal change near the sciatic notch, but often MRI is used to exclude other causes (disc disease, pelvic masses). For proximal hamstring tendinopathy, MRI shows thickening or partial tears at the hamstring origin, with possible bursal fluid under the ischial tuberosity. Standard hip MRI sequences (coronal T2, axial T2) often capture the relevant tendon pathology [28].

X-Ray Plain radiographs of the pelvis/hip are of limited use for soft tissue syndromes except to rule out bony causes. For example, an X-ray may show hip osteoarthritis (joint space narrowing, osteophytes), femoral neck stress fracture or FAI morphology (cam or pincer lesions). In an older adult with lateral hip pain, an AP pelvis X-ray is often obtained to exclude severe arthrosis or subchondral fracture. However, radiographs are typically normal in isolated soft tissue conditions.

Overall, imaging should complement clinical assessment: in suspected gluteal tendinopathy, the combination of ultrasound or MRI findings (tendon abnormality) with the typical exam clinches the diagnosis.

Management [29, 8, 21]

Management of hip and pelvic girdle soft tissue syndromes is largely *conservative* with gradual escalation. The mainstays are the following:

- *Activity modification*: Avoid or limit activities that provoke symptoms (e.g. lying on the affected side for GTPS, deep squatting for hamstring, prolonged sitting for piriformis). Gradual return as tolerated.
- *Non-steroidal anti-inflammatory drugs (NSAIDs)*: Used for pain control. Although true inflammation is often minimal (tendinopathy is degenerative), NSAIDs can relieve discomfort for GTPS and iliopsoas syndromes.
- *Physiotherapy*: A tailored exercise program is crucial. Typical components include the following:
  - *Strengthening*: Focus on hip abductors (gluteus medius/minimus), hip extensors, core stabilisers and hamstrings, depending on syndrome. For GTPS, start with low-level isometrics progressing to resisted abduction and lower limb strengthening; for hamstring tendinopathy, emphasise eccentric hamstring loading.
  - *Biomechanical training*: Gait training (address limp or Trendelenburg), core stabilisation and correcting leg-length or pelvic alignment issues. Patients with hip tendinopathies often benefit from neuromuscular training to improve single-leg stance control.
- *Supportive measures*: Ice or heat packs as needed. Use of cushions or pillows to offload pressure on the trochanteric or ischial areas. Proper footwear or orthotics if biomechanical foot issues contribute.

Many patients experience significant improvement with these conservative measures. However, recovery may take several months, particularly for chronic gluteal or proximal hamstring tendinopathy. Gradual progression of load is key to avoid symptom flare.

Image-Guided Injections If pain persists despite rehab, or if rapid relief is needed, targeted injections can be employed:

- *Trochanteric bursa injections*: Ultrasound-guided corticosteroid (often with anaesthetic) injection into the trochanteric bursa or subgluteus medius bursa is common for GTPS. Short-term pain relief is typical, but effectiveness wanes after a few months [12]. Note that corticosteroid injections target the bursal inflammation; for gluteal tendinopathy, peritendinous injection (just under the tendon) may improve outcomes.
- *Iliopsoas bursal injections*: Ultrasound- or fluoroscopy-guided injection at the lesser trochanter/anterior hip can relieve iliopsoas tendinitis. These injections are also used diagnostically (pain relief confirms diagnosis).
- *Hamstring origin injection*: Injection of local steroid/anaesthetic around the ischial tuberosity tendon origin is occasionally used for proximal hamstring tendinopathy [25]. Care is taken to avoid intraneural injection.
- *Platelet-rich plasma (PRP)*: For chronic tendinopathies (gluteal, hamstring), PRP injections are offered by some, although evidence is still emerging. A systematic review suggests PRP may help gluteal tendinopathy, but high-quality trials are limited [16].

Extracorporeal Shock Wave Therapy (ESWT) Particularly for recalcitrant GTPS, low-energy ESWT has been shown in some trials to improve pain better than steroid injection at 1-year follow-up [17]. ESWT is less commonly used for other hip tendinopathies but can be considered if available.

Surgical Referral Most cases never require surgery. Indications for surgical referral include the following:

- Full-thickness gluteus medius/minimus tears causing persistent weakness and pain (can be repaired arthroscopically or via mini open approach)
- Refractory trochanteric bursitis not responding to injections/therapy (treated by bursectomy, IT band lengthening).
- Chronic proximal hamstring tears or ischial bursitis unresponsive to rehab (treated by debridement or tendon repair).
- Intractable iliopsoas tendinopathy after total hip arthroplasty (may need tendon release).

Surgery is reserved for severe and functionally limiting cases and patients should be counselled on the lengthy rehabilitation required postoperatively.

Prognosis and Prevention

Prognosis for soft tissue hip syndromes is generally favourable with appropriate treatment, but recovery often takes months. GTPS and iliopsoas syndromes, in particular, can be slow to resolve completely because tendons heal poorly. However, most patients eventually experience significant relief with conservative measures. Lustenberger et al. found symptom resolution in a substantial proportion of patients treated nonoperatively, and only 1–2 courses of injection or therapy were usually needed [17]. A prospective study of GTPS showed over 90% improvement with non-surgical management in many cohorts.

Recurrence is possible if underlying biomechanics are not corrected. Prevention focuses on addressing predisposing factors: maintaining strong hip abductors and core muscles, ensuring proper training techniques (especially in athletes), avoiding overuse and sudden increases in activity and controlling weight to reduce mechanical load. Stretching of the iliotibial band, hip flexors and hamstrings can help prevent tendon overload. In runners and sportspeople, gradual progression and cross-training reduce risk of tendinopathy. For patients with leg length discrepancy or pelvic tilt, orthotics or pelvic support may redistribute forces and prevent chronic strain [11].

As with other tendinopathies, complete rest is not advised (unless acute); rather, guided loading of the tendon promotes healing. Education about early symptom recognition is key so that intervention is started before severe degeneration occurs. In conclusion, with timely diagnosis and comprehensive management, most patients return to normal activities. Rare cases with late diagnosis or severe tendon tears may have persistent symptoms, underscoring the importance of holistic rehabilitation and preventive strategies.

Key Learning Points

- *GTPS commonly due to tendinopathy*: Lateral hip pain in older adults is most often caused by gluteus medius/minimus tendinopathy or tears, with only a minority having true trochanteric bursitis. Physical exam shows greater trochanter tenderness and pain on resisted hip abduction.
- *Differentiate from hip joint/spine*: Pain location and exam clues separate soft tissue vs joint or spine sources, for example, inability to put on shoes points to hip joint involvement, while pain below the knee with neurological signs suggests spine.
- *Imaging guides treatment*: Ultrasound/MRI are useful to confirm tendon tears or bursitis if needed, but normal imaging does not exclude clinical GTPS or piriformis syndrome. X-rays screen for arthritis or bony issues.
- *Conservative therapy first*: All these syndromes respond to a trial of rest/modification, physiotherapy (strength/stretch exercises) and NSAIDs. Injections (steroid/anaesthetic) into the relevant bursa or muscle can expedite relief for refractory pain.
- *Surgery rarely needed*: Endoscopic or open surgical repair (e.g. gluteal tendon repair, tendon release) is reserved for severe, persistent cases that fail exhaustive conservative care.
- *Prognosis*: With proper management, most patients improve over weeks to months. Preventive measures (strengthening, technique adjustment, weight control) help reduce recurrence.

References

1. Pianka MA, Serino J, DeFroda SF, Bodendorfer BM. Greater trochanteric pain syndrome: evaluation and management of a wide spectrum of pathology. SAGE Open Med. 2021;9:20503121211022584.Availablefrom:http://www.ncbi.nlm.nih.gov/pubmed/34158938.
2. Polkowski GG, Clohisy JC. Hip biomechanics. Sports Med Arthrosc. 2010;18(2):56–62. Available from: http://www.ncbi.nlm.nih.gov/pubmed/20473123.
3. Pumarejo Gomez L, Li D, Childress JM. Greater trochanteric pain syndrome (Greater trochanteric bursitis). StatPearls; 2026. Available from: http://www.ncbi.nlm.nih.gov/pubmed/26491621.
4. Flack NAMS, Nicholson HD, Woodley SJ. A review of the anatomy of the hip abductor muscles, gluteus medius, gluteus minimus, and tensor fascia lata. Clin Anat. 2012;25(6):697–708. Available from: http://www.ncbi.nlm.nih.gov/pubmed/22109658.
5. Sunil Kumar KH, Rawal J, Nakano N, Sarmento A, Khanduja V. Pathogenesis and contemporary diagnoses for lateral hip pain: a scoping review. Knee Surg Sports Traumatol Arthrosc. 2021;29(8):2408–16. Available from: http://www.ncbi.nlm.nih.gov/pubmed/33341914.
6. Lifshitz L, Bar Sela S, Gal N, Martin R, Fleitman KM. Iliopsoas the hidden muscle: anatomy, diagnosis, and treatment. Curr Sports Med Rep. 2020;19(6):235–43. Available from: http://www.ncbi.nlm.nih.gov/pubmed/32516195.
7. Chamberlain R. Hip pain in adults: evaluation and differential diagnosis. Am Fam Physician. 2021;103(2):81–9. Available from: http://www.ncbi.nlm.nih.gov/pubmed/33448767.
8. Hicks BL, Lam JC, Varacallo MA. Piriformis syndrome. StatPearls; 2026. Available from: http://www.ncbi.nlm.nih.gov/pubmed/30013870.
9. Linklater JM, Hamilton B, Carmichael J, Orchard J, Wood DG. Hamstring injuries: anatomy, imaging, and intervention. Semin Musculoskelet Radiol. 2010;14(2):131–61. Available from: http://www.ncbi.nlm.nih.gov/pubmed/20486024.
10. Gandbhir VN, Lam JC, Lui F, Rayi A. Trendelenburg Gait. StatPearls; 2026. Available from: http://www.ncbi.nlm.nih.gov/pubmed/9917586.
11. Santos LEN, Navarro TP, Machado CJ, de Cabrita HABA, Pires RE, Figueiredo LB, et al. Relationship of the pelvic-trochanteric index with greater trochanteric pain syndrome. Clinics (Sao Paulo). 2021;76:e3312. Available from: http://www.ncbi.nlm.nih.gov/pubmed/34852141.
12. Long SS, Surrey DE, Nazarian LN. Sonography of greater trochanteric pain syndrome and the rarity of primary bursitis. Am J Roentgenol. 2013;201(5):1083–6. Available from: https://www.ajronline.org/doi/10.2214/AJR.12.10038.
13. Silva F, Adams T, Feinstein J, Arroyo RA. Trochanteric bursitis: refuting the myth of inflammation. J Clin Rheumatol. 2008;14(2):82–6. Available from: http://www.ncbi.nlm.nih.gov/pubmed/18391678.
14. Poultsides LA, Bedi A, Kelly BT. An algorithmic approach to mechanical hip pain. HSS J. 2012;8(3):213–24. Available from: http://www.ncbi.nlm.nih.gov/pubmed/24082863.
15. Ladurner A, Fitzpatrick J, O'Donnell JM. Treatment of gluteal tendinopathy: a systematic review and stage-adjusted treatment recommendation. Orthop J Sport Med. 2021;9(7):23259671211016850. Available from: http://www.ncbi.nlm.nih.gov/pubmed/34377713.
16. Ahmed H, Tarar MY, Khalid A, Shah N, Gilani A, Ijaz M. Greater trochanteric pain syndrome and the efficacy of platelet-rich plasma injections: a systematic review. Cureus. 2024;16(10):e72597. Available from: http://www.ncbi.nlm.nih.gov/pubmed/39610638.
17. Lustenberger DP, Ng VY, Best TM, Ellis TJ. Efficacy of treatment of trochanteric bursitis: a systematic review. Clin J Sport Med. 2011;21(5):447–53. Available from: http://www.ncbi.nlm.nih.gov/pubmed/21814140
18. Johnston CA, Wiley JP, Lindsay DM, Wiseman DA. Iliopsoas bursitis and tendinitis. A review. Sports Med. 1998;25(4):271–83. Available from: http://www.ncbi.nlm.nih.gov/pubmed/9587184.

19. Vandeputte F-J, Driesen R, Timmermans A, Corten K. Evaluation of clinical tests to diagnose iliopsoas tendinopathy. Clin Orthop Relat Res. 2025;483(11):2123–32. Available from: http://www.ncbi.nlm.nih.gov/pubmed/40388705.
20. Bakhsh W, Childs S, Kenney R, Schiffman S, Giordano B. Iliopsoas snapping hip: improving the diagnostic value of magnetic resonance imaging with a novel parameter. Skeletal Radiol. 2019;48(6):889–96. Available from: http://www.ncbi.nlm.nih.gov/pubmed/30280202.
21. Anderson CN. Iliopsoas: pathology, diagnosis, and treatment. Clin Sports Med. 2016;35(3):419–33. Available from: http://www.ncbi.nlm.nih.gov/pubmed/27343394.
22. Nunley RM, Wilson JM, Gilula L, Clohisy JC, Barrack RL, Maloney WJ. Iliopsoas bursa injections can be beneficial for pain after total hip arthroplasty. Clin Orthop Relat Res. 2010;468(2):519–26. Available from: http://www.ncbi.nlm.nih.gov/pubmed/19851816.
23. Grimaldi A, Mellor R, Nasser A, Vicenzino B, Hunter DJ. Current and future advances in practice: tendinopathies of the hip. Rheumatol Adv Pract. 2024;8(2):rkae022. Available from: http://www.ncbi.nlm.nih.gov/pubmed/38601140.
24. Goom TSH, Malliaras P, Reiman MP, Purdam CR. Proximal hamstring tendinopathy: clinical aspects of assessment and management. J Orthop Sports Phys Ther. 2016;46(6):483–93. Available from: http://www.ncbi.nlm.nih.gov/pubmed/27084841.
25. Nasser AM, Vicenzino B, Grimaldi A, Anderson J, Semciw AI. Proximal hamstring tendinopathy: a systematic review of interventions. Int J Sports Phys Ther. 2021;16(2):288–305. Available from: http://www.ncbi.nlm.nih.gov/pubmed/33842025.
26. Raj MA, Ampat G, Varacallo MA. Sacroiliac joint pain. StatPearls; 2026. Available from: http://www.ncbi.nlm.nih.gov/pubmed/16244008.
27. Hutchinson LA, Lichtwark GA, Willy RW, Kelly LA. The iliotibial band: a complex structure with versatile functions. Sports Med. 2022;52(5):995–1008. Available from: http://www.ncbi.nlm.nih.gov/pubmed/35072941.
28. Mak MS, Teh J. Magnetic resonance imaging of the hip: anatomy and pathology. Polish J Radiol. 2020;85:e489–508. Available from: http://www.ncbi.nlm.nih.gov/pubmed/33101554.
29. Reid D. The management of greater trochanteric pain syndrome: a systematic literature review. J Orthop. 2016;13(1):15–28. Available from: http://www.ncbi.nlm.nih.gov/pubmed/26955229.

Knee: Tendons and Bursae

9

Abstract

Anterior knee pain related to tendons and bursae is a common presentation in both athletes and general practice. This chapter reviews knee tendon and bursal anatomy, biomechanics and typical overuse injuries affecting the patellar tendon, iliotibial band (ITB) and several knee bursae. We discuss clinical features of patellar tendinopathy ("jumper's knee"), ITB friction syndrome and bursitis of the pes anserinus, prepatellar, infrapatellar and suprapatellar regions. A differential diagnosis for anterior, lateral and medial knee pain is outlined. Key physical exam manoeuvres (e.g. Noble and Ober tests for ITB, resisted knee extension for patellar tendon, pes anserine palpation) are described. Imaging indications are discussed: ultrasound is excellent for visualising tendon degeneration or bursal fluid, X-ray for bone pathology (e.g. osteophytes, tibial tubercle ossicles or sequelae of Osgood-Schlatter disease) and MRI for complex or refractory cases. Management emphasises conservative care: activity modification, physiotherapy (eccentric loading for tendinopathy, hip abductor and core strengthening for ITB syndrome, periarticular strengthening for knee), NSAIDs, bracing or padding (knee strap, kneepad) and cryotherapy. Ultrasound-guided injections (corticosteroid for bursitis, regenerative injections for chronic tendinopathy) are indicated when simpler measures fail, with caution around tendon injections. Referral to sports medicine or orthopaedics is considered for frank tendon rupture, mechanical joint derangements or refractory symptoms. Understanding anatomy, exam and treatment options can improve outcomes in these often chronic knee soft tissue conditions.

Clinical Vignette

A 42-year-old male recreational basketball player presents with gradually worsening anterior knee pain for 6 months. He initially noted soreness at the lower pole of the kneecap after jumping, which now becomes a sharp ache when he ascends stairs or

© The Author(s), under exclusive license to Springer Nature Switzerland AG 2026

R. Amarnani, *Soft Tissue and Musculoskeletal Medicine in Rheumatology*,
https://doi.org/10.1007/978-3-032-29441-8_9

after prolonged sitting. On exam, he has point tenderness at the patellar tendon just below the patella and pain when doing a single-leg squat on a 25° decline board. There is no joint effusion or ligament instability. Ultrasound demonstrates a thickened, heterogeneous distal patellar tendon with increased neovascularity/power Doppler signal. He is diagnosed with patellar tendinopathy (jumper's knee) and advised on load management and eccentric leg strengthening exercises. He is given NSAIDs and a patellar strap. After 3 months of physiotherapy his pain is reduced but not resolved, so continued progressive loading is advised; PRP may be discussed if symptoms remain refractory after a longer period of structured rehabilitation.

Anatomy and Biomechanics of the Knee Tendons and Bursae

The knee's anterior soft tissues include the extensor mechanism: the quadriceps tendon (inserting on the patella) and the patellar tendon (continuing distally to the tibial tuberosity) [1]. These tendons transmit quadriceps force and stabilise the patella. The patellar tendon is particularly susceptible to repetitive loading injuries in athletes (Fig. 9.1). Laterally, the iliotibial band (ITB) is a thick fascia from the iliac crest (via tensor fasciae latae and gluteus maximus) inserting at Gerdy's tubercle on the anterolateral tibia [2] (Fig. 9.2). It functions as a dynamic lateral stabiliser of the knee, acting as a knee extensor near full extension and knee flexor beyond 30° [3]. Repetitive knee flexion-extension can increase compression and irritation of the tissues deep to the distal ITB around the lateral femoral epicondyle.

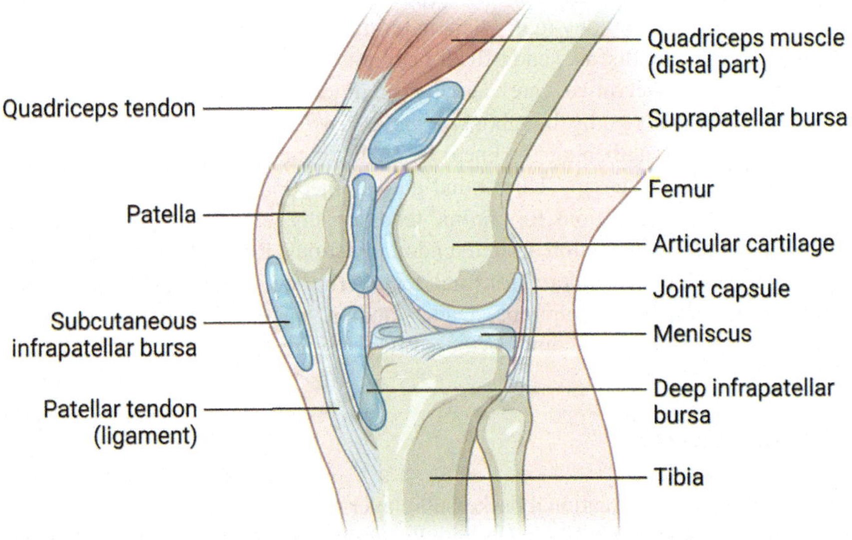

Fig. 9.1 Sagittal anatomy of the knee showing the quadriceps and patellar tendons and adjacent bursae

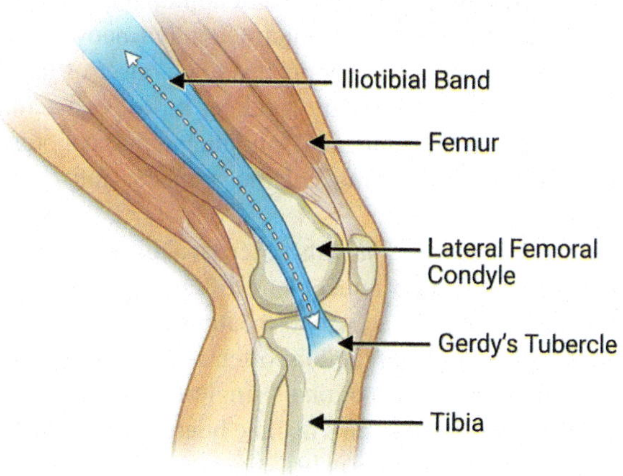

Fig. 9.2 Lateral view of the knee highlighting the iliotibial band's course

Bursae are fluid-filled sacs that reduce friction between moving tissues. The knee has several superficial bursae [4]: the *prepatellar bursa* (between skin and patella), *superficial infrapatellar bursa* (Clergyman's knee, between skin and patellar tendon) and *pes anserine bursa* (between the conjoined sartorius/gracilis/semitendinosus tendons and medial tibia). The *deep infrapatellar bursa* lies between the patellar tendon and tibial tubercle. A *suprapatellar bursa* (actually the suprapatellar pouch of the knee joint) lies above the patella and is continuous with the joint space.

Overlying the anteromedial proximal tibia, the pes anserine tendons (from sartorius, gracilis, semitendinosus) form a "goose's foot" near the knee [5]. The pes anserine bursa sits just beneath these tendons, facilitating smooth gliding. Deep to the quadriceps tendon, the *suprapatellar plica or bursa* can sometimes become inflamed, though this "bursa" is usually a knee joint recess and not an isolated sac.

Common Soft Tissue Conditions

Patellar Tendinopathy (Jumper's Knee)

Aetiology and Epidemiology Patellar tendinopathy is an overuse injury characterised by degenerative changes in the patellar tendon. It is common in sports with repetitive jumping or change of direction (e.g. volleyball, basketball) but can occur in recreational athletes and even inactive individuals [6]. Elite jumping athletes (volleyball, basketball) have prevalence rates up to ~45% [7]. Male sex and high-level sports participation (especially at the national level) are notable risk factors [8]. Other possible risks include taller or more active individuals, though data is mixed.

Pathophysiology [6] Patellar tendinopathy involves failed tendon healing with collagen disorganisation, microtears and neovascularity, rather than acute inflammation. Patients often report insidious onset of tendon pain at the inferior patellar pole, initially with activity and later more persistent. MRI and ultrasound typically show tendon thickening and inhomogeneous echotexture, sometimes with increased Doppler flow. Over time, calcific spurs can form within the tendon.

Clinical Features Patients describe aching or sharp anterior knee pain localised to the patellar tendon attachment, often worsening with jumping, squatting or prolonged sitting after activity ("theatre sign"). Examination reveals tenderness on palpation of the patellar tendon (often 1–2 cm below the patella) and pain with resisted knee extension. A functional "single-leg decline squat test" (having the patient perform a shallow squat on a decline board) will typically reproduce pain in the tendon, confirming the diagnosis [9].

Imaging Diagnosis is primarily clinical, but ultrasound can confirm tendon pathology (thickening, hypoechoic changes, Doppler signal). MRI shows tendon thickening and increased T2 signal in chronic cases [6]. Plain X-ray is usually unremarkable aside from possibly showing enthesophytes at the patella or tibial tubercle.

Treatment Non-operative treatment dominates [10]. Eccentric quadriceps exercises on a decline board are the mainstay. Other modalities include isometric strengthening, stretching of the quadriceps-hamstring complex and adjunctive therapies (cryotherapy, shockwave). Ankle, hip and core strengthening are also important to offload the tendon. Platelet-rich plasma (PRP) injections have shown some promise in refractory cases [10]. Corticosteroid injections are generally avoided in tendons due to weakening risk; if used, they are injected sparingly and often under ultrasound guidance. Surgery (tendon debridement or "stripping" of neovessels) is reserved for chronic nonresponders (taking often a year or more to recover).

Iliotibial Band Friction Syndrome

Aetiology and Epidemiology Iliotibial band syndrome (ITBS) is a common cause of lateral knee pain in runners and cyclists. It accounts for roughly 10% of running-related injuries and is the second most common knee problem in runners (after patellofemoral pain) [11]. Prevalence studies estimate 1.6–12% of runners develop ITBS [12]. Typical patients are endurance athletes (marathoners, triathletes, hikers) or cyclists. Women and novice runners may be at higher risk. Contributing factors include rapid increase in training volume, downhill running, leg length discrepancy, tight hip/leg musculature and poor biomechanics [11].

Pathophysiology The classical concept of "band friction" (the ITB rubbing over the lateral femoral epicondyle) has been questioned. Anatomical studies show the ITB has fibrous attachments that limit sliding, and instead a highly innervated fat pad beneath the ITB may be impinged during repeated knee flexion beyond 30° [11]. Regardless of exact mechanism, repetitive strain on the distal ITB leads to localised irritation around the lateral femoral epicondyle, and less commonly near the distal insertion at Gerdy's tubercle. ITBS presents as sharp or burning pain on the outside of the knee, typically worse at ~30° of flexion. Patients often report pain after running 2–4 miles, especially on inclines or uneven terrain. Pain may also occur when rising from a chair or descending stairs.

Clinical Features [13] On exam, there is point tenderness over the lateral femoral epicondyle or Gerdy's tubercle. The Noble compression test (patient supine, examiner applies pressure over the lateral epicondyle while passively extending the flexed knee) reproduces pain at ~30° flexion if ITBS is present. The Ober test (patient side-lying, hip flexed and abducted and then allowed to adduct) may reveal a tight ITB (inability of leg to drop to table level). Tightness of hip abductors or tensor fasciae latae on examination is common. Dynamic running or cycling gait analysis may show overpronation or poor hip control.

Imaging Imaging is not routinely required. MRI may show thickening of the distal ITB or fluid but is generally reserved for atypical cases or to rule out other lateral knee pathologies. X-rays are unremarkable unless advanced osteoarthritis is present. Ultrasound can identify lateral knee fluid or bursal swelling (a subtendinous bursa is sometimes present) but is not often used diagnostically for ITBS [2].

Treatment Conservative management is first line [14]. Focus is on load modification (reducing mileage, avoiding downhill runs), hip abductor and core strengthening (to improve mechanics), and correcting footwear or running form. NSAIDs and ice can help reduce inflammation. Recent evidence highlights the importance of hip abductor strengthening; a systematic review found that programmes incorporating hip abductor exercises (and possibly shockwave therapy) significantly improved ITBS symptoms [11]. Extracorporeal shockwave therapy (ESWT) has emerged as an adjunct for chronic cases [11]. Injection therapy (e.g. corticosteroid into the lateral bursa) is rarely used except in refractory ITBS or coexisting bursitis. Surgical lengthening of the ITB is rarely indicated today due to mixed outcomes.

Pes Anserine Bursitis

Aetiology and Epidemiology Pes anserine bursitis is an inflammation of the bursa under the pes anserinus tendons on the medial knee [5]. It commonly occurs in middle-aged women who are overweight or have knee osteoarthritis [15]. Because the pes anserine tendons form a broad insertion on the medial tibia, factors that increase knee valgus or tibial stress (e.g. pes planus feet, lateral thrust) can contribute. It can also follow medial knee injury or occur with overuse (running, jumping or climbing stairs).

Pathophysiology Chronic microtrauma from repetitive flexion (especially with valgus loading) irritates the pes anserine bursa [5]. Alternatively, acute trauma or direct blow may trigger bursitis, though more often symptoms are insidious.

Clinical Features [5] Patients report medial knee pain 5–7 cm below the joint line, often worse with climbing stairs or arising from a chair. They may describe tenderness at the pes anserinus area and possibly swelling. Physical exam shows point tenderness over the medial tibia just below the joint line; knee flexion or resisted internal rotation may provoke pain. There is usually no joint effusion or ligamentous laxity, distinguishing it from meniscal or MCL pathology. The condition overlaps with pes anserine "tendinopathy" (involving the tendons themselves) and both are sometimes called "pes anserine pain syndrome".

Imaging Plain radiographs of the knee are typically normal except for underlying OA. Ultrasound can show fluid distension of the bursa and is helpful for guided injection. MRI will demonstrate fluid and inflammation in the pes anserine region but is rarely needed if the diagnosis is clear.

Treatment Treatment is conservative. Weight loss and addressing OA (if present) are important. Physiotherapy focuses on strengthening the hip abductors and quadriceps to reduce valgus strain and stretching of the hamstrings. A medial knee strap or taping may offload the area. NSAIDs and ice reduce inflammation. If symptoms persist, an ultrasound-guided corticosteroid injection into the bursa can rapidly improve pain [16]. Pes anserine bursitis generally has a good prognosis with these measures.

Prepatellar Bursitis

Aetiology and Epidemiology Prepatellar bursitis ("housemaid's knee") is inflammation of the bursa overlying the patella [17]. It is common in occupations or activities involving frequent kneeling: floor layers, miners, gardeners and wrestlers. Acute trauma to the kneecap (direct blow or fall) can also cause it, as can repetitive microtrauma (like crawling). Septic prepatellar bursitis occurs when skin breaks (scratches, insect bites) introduce bacteria, often *Staphylococcus aureus*, into the bursa [18]. Patients with rheumatoid arthritis or gout are predisposed to aseptic bursitis at the knee.

Pathophysiology Chronic kneeling leads to constant pressure between the patella and skin, causing bursal irritation, fluid accumulation and thickening [17]. Infection produces an acutely inflamed, swollen bursa with warmth and possible systemic signs.

Clinical Features Patients present with anterior knee swelling over the patella. In noninfectious cases, the bursa is fluctuant but not overly painful unless moved. In septic bursitis, the bursa is tense, tender and red and fever may be present. Range of motion is usually preserved unless very swollen. Unlike patellar tendon injury, the extensor mechanism is intact.

Imaging X-rays are usually unremarkable (used to exclude bony injury). Ultrasound can confirm fluid in the prepatellar bursa and guide aspiration if needed. MRI is rarely needed except if deep infection or underlying pathology (e.g. patellar fracture) is suspected.

Treatment [17] Initial management follows general bursitis principles: avoid kneeling and irritation, use knee pads, apply ice and use NSAIDs. In aseptic cases that do not resolve, aspiration of the fluid can relieve tension. For septic bursitis, oral or intravenous antibiotics (covering *Staph*/*Strep*) are started promptly; hospitalised intravenous therapy is indicated for severe infection. Aspiration and culturing of bursal fluid is mandatory if infection is suspected. Recalcitrant noninfectious bursitis may require surgical bursectomy, but this is rare.

Other Bursal Inflammation (Infrapatellar, Suprapatellar)

The *superficial infrapatellar bursa* lies over the patellar tendon just below the patella (sometimes called Clergyman's knee) [4]. It, too, can become inflamed from kneeling, though it is much less common than prepatellar bursitis. Patients have pain and swelling just below the patella over the tendon. Management is similar to prepatellar bursitis (padding, NSAIDs, aspiration/steroid if needed).

The *deep infrapatellar bursa* (between the patellar tendon and tibial tuberosity) may be implicated in Osgood-Schlatter disease (in adolescents) or in adults after patellar tendon injury. It can cause anterior knee pain on kneeling, but isolated deep infrapatellar bursitis is uncommon.

The so-called *suprapatellar bursa* is actually a synovial recess of the knee joint. Fluid distension of this pouch ("suprapatellar effusion") can occur with intraarticular pathology (e.g. meniscus tear, arthritis) or rarely with inflammatory bursitis. True isolated suprapatellar bursitis is unusual, but pain or swelling just above the patella should prompt evaluation for joint effusion or synovial disorders [1].

Differential Diagnosis of Anterior, Lateral and Medial Knee Pain

Anterior Knee Pain [19] Patellofemoral pain syndrome (chondromalacia patellae) is very common, especially in adolescents and young adults with maltracking; it causes pain around or behind the patella exacerbated by squatting, stair climbing or prolonged sitting. Other anterior causes include quadriceps tendinopathy (pain at the superior patellar pole), Osgood-Schlatter disease (tibial tubercle apophysitis in adolescents), Sinding-Larsen-Johansson syndrome (apophysitis of inferior patella), patellar subluxation or dislocation, patellar stress fracture, Hoffa's fat pad impingement and prepatellar bursitis. Referred pain from the hip or lumbar spine should also be considered. In an older adult, osteoarthritis (particularly patellofemoral osteoarthritis) can manifest as anterior knee pain.

Lateral Knee Pain [20] The differential includes iliotibial band syndrome (pain over the lateral femoral condyle), lateral meniscus tear (pain/clicking with twisting, joint line tenderness), lateral collateral ligament sprain, popliteus tendinopathy (posterolateral knee pain, especially when downhill running), fibular head bursitis and osteoarthritis of the lateral compartment. Peroneal nerve irritation at the knee can mimic lateral pain. Patellofemoral syndrome can also cause lateral pain if the patella is tracking laterally. Rarely, referred pain from the lateral hip or sciatic nerve can be perceived at the knee. Common causes listed include ITBS, lateral compartment arthritis, popliteus tendonitis, LCL/PCL sprain and meniscus injury.

Medial Knee Pain [21] Consider pes anserine bursitis (point tenderness inferomedially), medial meniscus tear (joint line pain, clicking/locking, pain on twisting or McMurray's test), medial collateral ligament (MCL) sprain (acute trauma with valgus force), medial plica syndrome and osteoarthritis of the medial compartment. Infrapatellar bursitis can cause pain just below the patella. Systemic conditions (gout, RA) often involve the medial knee via joint or bursae. A thorough history/exam distinguishes these: for example, an MCL injury usually follows a known pivot injury, whereas pes bursitis often occurs insidiously in an overweight patient. Referred pain from the ipsilateral hip (e.g. trochanteric bursitis) should also be on the differential.

Physical Examination and Key Provocative Tests [22]

A careful knee exam begins with inspection (swelling, erythema, alignment) and palpation. In anterior knee pain, palpate the patellar tendon and quadriceps tendon for tenderness or thickening. The *painful arc test* (pain during active knee flexion/extension) is nonspecific but noted. Patellofemoral compression (Clarke's) test can reproduce PFPS pain (patella grind). The *single-leg decline squat* on a 25° board can provoke patellar tendinopathy. For ITB syndrome, the *Noble compression test* is performed with the patient supine and knee flexed ~90°. The examiner applies firm thumb pressure just above the lateral femoral condyle while passively extending the knee; pain at ~30° confirms ITB irritation. The *Ober test* (patient side-lying; examiner extends the hip and adducts the leg from an abducted position) assesses ITB tightness (positive if the lower leg cannot drop to table level) [11]. Pain with resisted hip abduction or external rotation can also indicate ITB or TFL tightness.

For medial knee, palpate the pes anserinus (just below the medial joint line about 5–7 cm from it) for tenderness. Resisted knee flexion (especially against internal tibial rotation) may aggravate pes symptoms. MCL stability is tested with valgus stress at 0° and 30° flexion. Joint line tenderness may indicate meniscal tear; the McMurray test or Thessaly test (patient standing on one leg with slight knee bend while internally/externally rotating) can reproduce meniscal pain. Infrapatellar bursitis yields tenderness just below the patella. For suprapatellar assessment, look for suprapatellar effusion (bulging of the pouch) with the "patellar tap" or "sweep test".

General knee exam should also check ligament stability (Lachman, anterior/posterior drawer), popliteal fossa, foot and hip. Gait, squat mechanics and lower limb alignment (Q-angle, varus/valgus) are informative for biomechanical contributions.

Imaging: When to Use Ultrasound, X-Ray and MRI

X-Ray Start with plain radiographs if bony pathology is a concern. AP and lateral knee films can reveal osteoarthritis, Osgood-Schlatter lesions (tibial tubercle apophysitis), bipartite patella, stress fractures, loose bodies or patellar malalignment. In soft tissue pain with a normal exam, X-ray is often unremarkable, but it remains useful in initial evaluation and ruling out arthropathy.

Ultrasound [23] Ultrasound is excellent for evaluating superficial soft tissues. It can visualise tendon structure (thickening, hypoechoic areas, neovessels) and bursal fluid or synovitis. For example, a tender patellar tendon can be scanned to confirm tendinopathy. The Achilles and patellar tendons are particularly amenable to high-resolution ultrasound. Ultrasound also guides diagnostic or therapeutic injections into bursae or around tendons. When bursitis is suspected (prepatellar, infrapatellar, pes), ultrasound will show an anechoic or hypoechoic fluid collection. It can distinguish a tense bursal fluid from adjacent soft tissue oedema. Thus, point-of-care ultrasound is often used by rheumatologists or sports medicine physicians to confirm bursitis or tendinitis and to guide needle placement.

MRI [24] MRI is more expensive but provides comprehensive assessment of the knee. It should be considered if initial management fails, if the diagnosis is unclear, or if a complex lesion is suspected. MRI clearly shows tendon tears, partial thickness lesions, bone marrow oedema and meniscal or cartilage injuries that might mimic tendon pain. For example, persistent anterior knee pain unresponsive to therapy may warrant MRI to look for patellar tendon partial tear or osteochondral defects. MRI is also useful when suspecting joint or synovial disease (e.g. synovitis, pigmented villonodular synovitis) or deep bursitis (suprapatellar pouch effusion).

In summary, ultrasound is the first choice for suspected tendon or bursal pathology (due to convenience and cost), while X-ray and MRI are used to rule out or confirm other intraarticular or bony causes when indicated.

Conservative Management: Physiotherapy, NSAIDs, Bracing and Activity Modification [25]

Initial management of tendinopathy and bursitis is non-operative. *Physiotherapy* is key: tailored exercise programmes address specific deficits. In patellar tendinopathy, progressive eccentric (or heavy slow) loading of the quadriceps strongly helps tendon remodelling. Hip and core strengthening (especially gluteus medius/abductors) improve leg alignment for both patellar and ITB syndromes. Stretching tight structures (quadriceps, hamstrings, ITB, hip flexors) relieves abnormal stresses. Balance and proprioceptive training around the knee can also be beneficial. For pes anserine bursitis, strengthening the vastus medialis and gluteal muscles is helpful, and weight loss is advised if overweight.

Bracing and taping may provide symptomatic relief. A patellar strap (placed over the patellar tendon below the kneecap) can unload the tendon in jumper's knee. Knee sleeves or braces that offload the joint (valgus braces) can reduce medial knee stress. For ITB, kinesiology tape or a strap around the distal thigh can sometimes reduce tension. Kneepads or wedge insoles are recommended for those with knee pain on kneeling (prepatellar or infrapatellar bursitis).

NSAIDs and Analgesics Short-term NSAIDs or paracetamol are often used to control pain and inflammation. For acute bursitis flares or tendinitis, a brief course of NSAIDs may be reasonable. Cryotherapy (ice) applied 3–4 times daily for 15–20 min can help acute swelling.

Activity Modification Crucial to identify and avoid inciting activities. Runners with patellar or ITB issues should reduce mileage, avoid hills or uneven terrain and cross-train (swimming, cycling) until symptoms improve. Athletes may temporarily switch to low-impact sports. Ergonomic changes (footwear, orthotics for genu valgum) can be implemented. Occupational patients (roofers, gardeners) should use knee pads and take frequent breaks. Patient education on gradually returning to activity with pain-guided limits is emphasised.

Injection Therapy: Indications and Guidance [26]

Injection therapies are considered for patients who fail an adequate course of conservative care (often 3–6 months). *Corticosteroid injections* are commonly used for bursitis and less often for tendinopathy. For example, a corticosteroid injection into the pes anserine bursa or prepatellar bursa can quickly relieve pain and inflammation when physiotherapy and NSAIDs have not worked. The injection is usually performed under ultrasound guidance to help ensure accurate placement and reduce the risk of inadvertent intratendinous injection.

Cautions: Corticosteroids can weaken tendon tissue, so they are used sparingly around tendons. In patellar tendinopathy, steroid injections are generally avoided or limited to small volumes, as they may worsen tendon degeneration or risk rupture. If steroid is used for tendon, ultrasound is recommended to avoid intratendinous injection. For ITBS, steroid injection into a lateral subtendinous bursa (if present) or around the band can be tried, but long-term efficacy is unclear.

Regenerative Injections Platelet-rich plasma (PRP) and prolotherapy (hyperosmolar dextrose) have gained popularity for chronic tendinopathy. Some evidence (albeit limited) suggests PRP may improve long-term outcomes in jumper's knee better than steroid [6]. These are still considered experimental by many rheumatologists. High-volume saline injections ("needling" without drugs) under ultrasound have been explored in patellar tendon as well.

Ultrasound Guidance Whenever precise placement is important (e.g. small bursa, deep tendon or avoiding neurovascular structures), ultrasound guidance improves accuracy and reduces complications. Guidance is especially recommended for injections around the iliotibial band, the medial pes anserine region (to avoid the saphenous nerve) and intraarticular injections. For superficial bursae, blind injection can sometimes be done but US guidance minimises risk of intratendinous injection.

Other Injections Rarely, viscosupplementation (hyaluronic acid) injections have been tried in knee bursitis, but evidence is lacking. Botulinum toxin injection into the vastus medialis has been studied for refractory patellar pain, but this is not routine.

In summary, injection therapy is an adjunct: corticosteroid for recalcitrant bursitis or tendon sheath inflammation and PRP or similar for chronic tendinopathy when patients have not responded to rehab. Always evaluate for infection before injecting a bursa.

When to Refer to Orthopaedics or Sports Medicine

Most knee tendon and bursal problems can be managed in primary care or sports medicine. Referral is indicated for red flags or treatment failure. *Red flags* include signs of septic bursitis (high fever, intense erythema, purulent aspirate), which require urgent orthopaedic evaluation; suspicion of a quadriceps or complete patellar tendon rupture (inability to actively extend the knee or palpable tendon gap), which is a surgical emergency; or major joint derangements (loose bodies, large meniscal tears causing mechanical locking).

Chronic cases not responding to 6–12 months of conservative management warrant specialty referral. For example, an athlete whose patellar tendinopathy fails eccentric therapy and injection may be referred for consideration of surgical debridement or advanced treatments (arthroscopic shaving of tendon). Similarly, persistent ITB syndrome despite thorough biomechanical correction might be evaluated for potential surgical release (rare). Patients with significant osteoarthritis revealed on imaging (contributing to knee pain) should see orthopaedics for discussion of medical vs surgical management.

Referral to a sports medicine specialist can also be useful for guided rehabilitation programmes, gait analysis or ultrasound-guided injection and diagnostic ultrasound if in doubt.

Prognosis and Prevention

The prognosis for most knee tendon and bursitis conditions is generally good with appropriate treatment, but recovery can be slow (months). Patellar tendinopathy can take 6–12 months to resolve [6]. ITB syndrome usually improves with load adjustment and rehab over weeks to months. Pes anserine and prepatellar bursitis often resolve completely with conservative measures, unless complicated by chronic joint disease. Recurrence is common if underlying risk factors (technique, obesity, kneeling habits) are not addressed.

Prevention Preventing recurrence involves correcting biomechanical and occupational factors. For tendinopathy, a gradual training programme with cross-training reduces overload. Hip strengthening and maintaining flexibility are preventive. Athletes should warm up properly and avoid sudden mileage increases. Knee pads should be worn for professions involving kneeling to prevent prepatellar and infrapatellar bursitis. Weight management and gait analysis may help those prone to medial knee pain. Regular stretching of the ITB, proper shoe wear and running form coaching can prevent ITBS. In patients with rheumatoid arthritis or gout, optimal disease control reduces bursitis risk.

Prognosis is best when diagnosis and treatment are timely. Educating patients on their condition and proper mechanics often leads to sustained improvement. Long-term outcomes improve when patients follow a structured rehab and avoid repeat injury.

Key Learning Points

- *Anatomy*: The knee has several superficial bursae (prepatellar, infrapatellar, pes anserine) and key tendons (quadriceps/patellar, iliotibial band) that can be inflamed by repetitive stress.
- *Patellar tendinopathy*: Presents as anterior knee pain in jumpers; diagnosed clinically, confirmed by ultrasound/MRI; and treated with eccentric quadriceps exercises, load management and rarely injections.
- *Iliotibial band syndrome*: Lateral knee pain in runners/cyclists; positive Noble's test and Ober's test; treat with ITB stretching, hip abductor strengthening and shockwave therapy.
- *Pes anserine bursitis*: Medial knee pain in overweight women or those with knee OA; tender 5–7 cm below medial joint line; treat conservatively with rehab and NSAIDs and steroid injection if needed.
- *Prepatellar bursitis*: Anterior knee swelling from kneeling or trauma; manage with rest, ice, NSAIDs and padding; aspirate if diagnosis is uncertain, tense or infection is suspected; treat infection urgently. Corticosteroid injection should be used cautiously and only after infection has been excluded.
- *Physical exam*: Localise tenderness (patellar tendon vs joint line vs pes anserine). Use specific tests: Noble compression for ITB, single-leg decline squat for patellar tendon and resisted knee flexion for pes anserine. Always assess ligament stability to rule out MCL/LCL injury.
- *Imaging*: Use X-ray to exclude fractures or arthritis; ultrasound for real-time tendon/bursal assessment and guided injection; and MRI for complex or refractory cases.
- *Management*: Begin with conservative measures (activity modification, physiotherapy, knee pads, NSAIDs). Guided steroid injections for persistent bursitis; PRP or other regenerative injections for chronic tendinopathies. Referral if tendon rupture, mechanical joint pathology or failure of conservative therapy.
- *Prevention*: Encourage cross-training, proper biomechanics and protective padding to reduce repetitive stress. Early intervention and gradual training reduce chronicity of knee tendon and bursal injuries.

References

1. Flandry F, Hommel G. Normal anatomy and biomechanics of the knee. Sports Med Arthrosc [Internet]. 2011;19(2):82–92. Available from: http://www.ncbi.nlm.nih.gov/pubmed/21540705.
2. Hutchinson LA, Lichtwark GA, Willy RW, Kelly LA. The iliotibial band: a complex structure with versatile functions. Sports Med [Internet]. 2022;52(5):995–1008. Available from: http://www.ncbi.nlm.nih.gov/pubmed/35072941.
3. Gupton M, Imonugo O, Black AC, Launico MV, Terreberry RR. Anatomy, bony pelvis and lower limb. Knee [Internet] StatPearls. 2023; Available from: https://www.ncbi.nlm.nih.gov/books/NBK500017/.
4. Hasan M, Berkovich Y, Khatib M, Steinfeld Y, Sleiman A, Ben Zvi L, et al. Knee Bursae: a comprehensive review of clinical evaluation, imaging differentiation, and the expanding role of biologic therapies. Cartilage [Internet]. 2025:19476035251362430. Available from: http://www.ncbi.nlm.nih.gov/pubmed/41239892.
5. Mohseni M, Mabrouk A, Li D. Pes Anserine Bursitis [Internet]. StatPearls. 2024; Available from: https://www.ncbi.nlm.nih.gov/books/NBK532941/
6. Theodorou A, Komnos G, Hantes M. Patellar tendinopathy: an overview of prevalence, risk factors, screening, diagnosis, treatment and prevention. Arch Orthop Trauma Surg [Internet]. 2023;143(11):6695–705. Available from: http://www.ncbi.nlm.nih.gov/pubmed/37542006.
7. Lian ØB, Engebretsen L, Bahr R. Prevalence of jumper's knee among elite athletes from different sports: a cross-sectional study. Am J Sports Med [Internet]. 2005;33(4):561–7. Available from: https://journals.sagepub.com/doi/10.1177/0363546504270454.
8. van der Worp H, van Ark M, Roerink S, Pepping G-J, van den Akker-Scheek I, Zwerver J. Risk factors for patellar tendinopathy: a systematic review of the literature. Br J Sports Med [Internet]. 2011;45(5):446–52. Available from: http://www.ncbi.nlm.nih.gov/pubmed/21367808.
9. Rath E, Schwarzkopf R, Richmond JC. Clinical signs and anatomical correlation of patellar tendinitis. Indian J Orthop [Internet]. 2010;44(4):435–7. Available from: http://www.ncbi.nlm.nih.gov/pubmed/20924486.
10. Arner JW, Kaeding CC, Bradley JP. Management of Patellar Tendinopathy. Arthroscopy [Internet]. 2024;40(1):13–5. Available from: http://www.ncbi.nlm.nih.gov/pubmed/38123261.
11. Hadeed A, Tapscott DC. Iliotibial band friction syndrome [Internet]. StatPearls. 2026; Available from: http://www.ncbi.nlm.nih.gov/pubmed/22147711
12. Sanchez-Alvarado A, Bokil C, Cassel M, Engel T. Effects of conservative treatment strategies for iliotibial band syndrome on pain and function in runners: a systematic review. Front Sport Act living [Internet]. 2024;6:1386456. Available from: http://www.ncbi.nlm.nih.gov/pubmed/39247483.
13. Lavine R. Iliotibial band friction syndrome. Curr Rev Musculoskelet Med [Internet] 2010 Jul 20;3(1–4):18–22. Available from: http://www.ncbi.nlm.nih.gov/pubmed/21063495.
14. Friede MC, Innerhofer G, Fink C, Alegre LM, Csapo R. Conservative treatment of iliotibial band syndrome in runners: are we targeting the right goals? Phys Ther Sport [Internet]. 2022;54:44–52. Available from: http://www.ncbi.nlm.nih.gov/pubmed/35007886.
15. Clapp A, Trecek J, Joyce M, Sundaram M. Pes anserine bursitis. Orthopedics [Internet]. 2008;31(4):306, 407–8. Available from: http://www.ncbi.nlm.nih.gov/pubmed/18453164.
16. Gouda W, Abbas AS, Abdel-Aziz TM, Shoaeir MZ, Ahmed W, Moshrif A, et al. Comparing the efficacy of local corticosteroid injection, platelet-rich plasma, and extracorporeal shockwave therapy in the treatment of pes anserine bursitis: a prospective, randomized, comparative study. Adv Orthop [Internet]. 2023;2023:5545520. Available from: http://www.ncbi.nlm.nih.gov/pubmed/37810418.
17. Rishor-Olney CR, Taqi M, Pozun A. Prepatellar bursitis [Internet]. StatPearls. 2026. Available from: http://www.ncbi.nlm.nih.gov/pubmed/24305696.
18. Truong J, Mabrouk A, Ashurst JV. Septic Bursitis [Internet]. StatPearls. 2026. Available from: http://www.ncbi.nlm.nih.gov/pubmed/30479679.

19. D'Ambrosi R, Meena A, Raj A, Ursino N, Hewett TE. Anterior Knee Pain: State of the Art. Sport Med – open [Internet]. 2022;8(1):98. Available from: http://www.ncbi.nlm.nih.gov/pubmed/35907139.
20. van de Water ATM. Lateral knee pain requires a thorough assessment and adequate, best-practice intervention. Int J Ther Massage Bodywork [Internet]. 2015;8(1):31–2. Available from: http://www.ncbi.nlm.nih.gov/pubmed/25780473.
21. Laprade RF, Wijdicks CA. The management of injuries to the medial side of the knee. J Orthop Sports Phys Ther [Internet]. 2012;42(3):221–33. Available from: http://www.ncbi.nlm.nih.gov/pubmed/22382986.
22. Rossi R, Dettoni F, Bruzzone M, Cottino U, D'Elicio DG, Bonasia DE. Clinical examination of the knee: know your tools for diagnosis of knee injuries. Sports Med Arthrosc Rehabil Ther Technol [Internet]. 2011;3:25. Available from: http://www.ncbi.nlm.nih.gov/pubmed/22035381.
23. Jacobson JA, Ruangchaijatuporn T, Khoury V, Magerkurth O. Ultrasound of the knee: common pathology excluding extensor mechanism. Semin Musculoskelet Radiol [Internet]. 2017;21(2):102–12. Available from: http://www.ncbi.nlm.nih.gov/pubmed/28355674.
24. Chien A, Weaver JS, Kinne E, Omar I. Magnetic resonance imaging of the knee. Polish J Radiol [Internet]. 2020;85:e509–31. Available from: http://www.ncbi.nlm.nih.gov/pubmed/33101555.
25. Duong V, Oo WM, Ding C, Culvenor AG, Hunter DJ. Evaluation and treatment of knee pain: a review. JAMA [Internet]. 2023;330(16):1568–80. Available from: http://www.ncbi.nlm.nih.gov/pubmed/37874571.
26. Poliwoda S, Noor N, Mousa B, Sarwary Z, Noss B, Urits I, et al. A comprehensive review of intraarticular knee injection therapy, geniculate injections, and peripheral nerve stimulation for knee pain in clinical practice. Orthop Rev (Pavia) [Internet]. 2022;14(4):38676. Available from: http://www.ncbi.nlm.nih.gov/pubmed/36267543.

10 Foot and Ankle Soft Tissue Conditions

Abstract

Foot and ankle soft tissue conditions cause significant morbidity and include common problems such as Achilles tendinopathy, plantar fasciitis, posterior tibial tendon dysfunction, peroneal tendinopathy and retrocalcaneal bursitis. These disorders often mimic systemic disease but are usually mechanical, degenerative tendinosis rather than true inflammatory processes. For example, plantar fasciitis usually reflects degenerative fasciopathy at the medial calcaneal origin rather than acute inflammation. Key anatomical and biomechanical factors (Achilles tendon insertion, plantar fascia arch support) are reviewed to ground understanding. Examination focuses on palpation of tendons and entheses, resisted muscle testing, gait and functional tests (e.g., single-leg heel raise, Windlass test). Imaging (X-ray, ultrasound, MRI) is guided by chronicity and differential. Management emphasises conservative care (rest, stretching, physiotherapy, orthotics) and judicious use of pain relief. Ultrasound-guided injections or extracorporeal shockwave/PRP are considered after failed initial therapy. Indications for referral (surgery) are highlighted. This chapter provides a practical approach to distinguishing and treating common foot/ankle soft tissue disorders in rheumatology practice, with attention to differentiating enthesitis and structural deformity from inflammatory arthropathies.

Clinical Vignette

A 45-year-old active woman presents with a 3-month history of right heel pain. She is an avid runner and describes sharp pain at the bottom of her heel that is worst with her first steps in the morning or after prolonged sitting, improving somewhat with walking. She denies fever, joint swelling or systemic symptoms. On exam, the right heel shows localised tenderness at the medial calcaneal tubercle (plantar fascia insertion) and tight calf muscles; ankle range-of-motion and neurovascular exam

© The Author(s), under exclusive license to Springer Nature Switzerland AG 2026

R. Amarnani, *Soft Tissue and Musculoskeletal Medicine in Rheumatology*,
https://doi.org/10.1007/978-3-032-29441-8_10

are normal. There is no significant hindfoot valgus or forefoot deformity. These findings are most consistent with plantar fasciitis (a degenerative enthesopathy), prompting conservative management with plantar stretching, heel support and activity modification.

Anatomy and Biomechanics

The foot and ankle have a complex anatomy that enables weight-bearing and propulsion [1]. The Achilles (calcaneal) tendon is the common tendon of the gastrocnemius and soleus muscles, inserting onto the posterior calcaneus. A fluid-filled *retrocalcaneal bursa* lies deep to the insertion, cushioning the tendon against the bone (Fig. 10.1). The Achilles tendon has a "watershed" zone of relatively poor blood supply approximately 2–6 cm proximal to the insertion [2], which is the typical site of mid-portion tendinopathy.

The plantar fascia is a thick aponeurosis originating at the medial calcaneal tubercle and fanning out towards the metatarsal heads. It comprises three bands that support the medial and lateral longitudinal arches and act as a dynamic shock absorber during gait [3]. During toe-off, the plantar fascia tightens in the *windlass mechanism*, helping to stabilise the arch.

The posterior tibial tendon passes behind the medial malleolus and inserts primarily onto the navicular tuberosity, with expansions to the cuneiforms, cuboid and bases of the second to fourth metatarsals. It is the main dynamic support of the

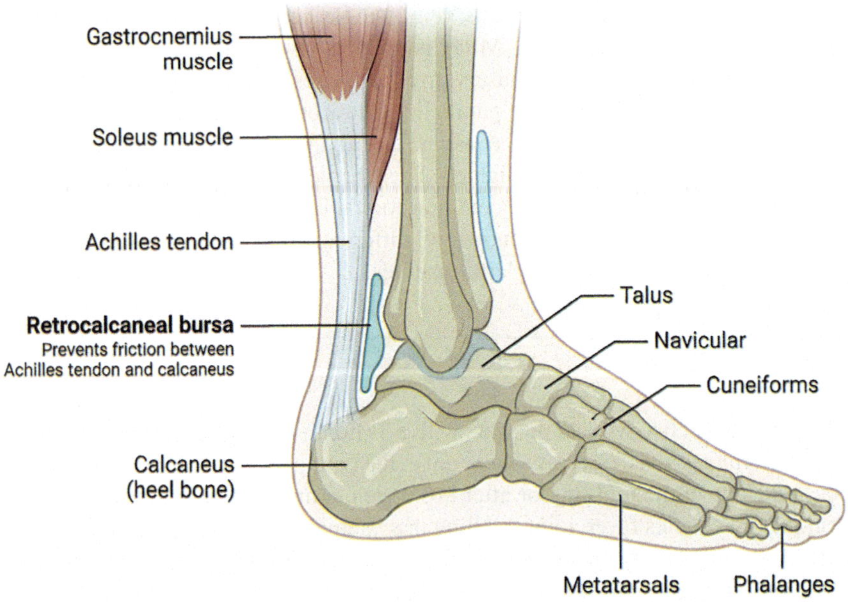

Fig. 10.1 Anatomy of the Achilles tendon and retrocalcaneal bursa

medial longitudinal arch, inverting and plantarflexing the foot [4]. The peroneus longus and brevis tendons run behind the lateral malleolus and evert the foot (longus to the first metatarsal/medial cuneiform, brevis to the base of the fifth metatarsal).

Normal biomechanics involve heel strike (calcaneus load), foot flattening at mid-stance (arch absorbs load) and push-off (Achilles and calf propel the body forward) [5]. A stable arch and normal tendon function allow even distribution of stress. Flatfoot (pes planus) or high-arched (pes cavus) deformities alter this load-sharing and can predispose to overuse injuries of the plantar fascia, Achilles or tibialis posterior tendon.

Common Soft Tissue Conditions

Achilles Tendinopathy

Achilles tendinopathy is a degenerative disorder of the calcaneal tendon. It is classified as mid-portion (2–6 cm proximal to insertion) or insertional (at the calcaneus) [2]. Mid-portion Achilles tendinosis is common in runners and jumpers. Insertional tendinopathy often coexists with retrocalcaneal bursitis or a Haglund's deformity (a bony prominence on the posterior calcaneus) [6]. Histologically, both forms are characterised by collagen degeneration and fibroblast proliferation, with few inflammatory cells.

Patients typically report activity-related heel pain (aches or burning), worse with exercise and often stiff after rest. Risk factors include repetitive overloading (especially sudden increases in training), limited ankle dorsiflexion, obesity, flatfoot or hindfoot malalignment and systemic factors such as diabetes or rheumatoid arthritis. Certain medications (fluoroquinolone antibiotics, systemic corticosteroids, statins) can predispose to tendon degeneration [7]. On exam, there is tenderness of the Achilles tendon (insertional pain may be more posterior and tender to palpation of the bursa). Pain may increase with resisted plantarflexion or during a single-leg heel raise.

Plantar Fasciitis

Plantar fasciitis is a degenerative overload injury of the plantar fascia at its origin on the medial calcaneus [8]. It is the most common cause of inferior heel pain. Patients (often ages 40–60) describe sharp heel pain with the first steps in the morning or after prolonged sitting, with gradual improvement after walking but recurrence of pain later in the day. Aggravating activities include running, jumping or prolonged standing on hard surfaces.

Predisposing factors are pes planus (flat feet) or pes cavus (high arches), tight gastrocnemius/soleus muscles (limited ankle dorsiflexion), obesity and occupations requiring prolonged standing or walking [9]. About 50% of patients may have a heel spur on X-ray, but this is not causative. Examination reveals point tenderness at the medial calcaneal tubercle (origin of the fascia), and sometimes a "windlass test" (pain on passive dorsiflexion of the great toe) is positive. Patients improve with conservative measures in most cases, although symptoms can persist for months [8].

Posterior Tibial Tendinopathy

Posterior tibial tendinopathy (tibialis posterior tendinosis or dysfunction) is a frequent cause of adult-acquired flatfoot deformity. It commonly affects middle-aged adults (especially obese women) and is often bilateral. It is strongly associated with systemic factors like hypertension, diabetes and collagen vascular disease but is fundamentally an overuse tendinopathy of the PTT [4]. Patients report medial ankle and arch pain that worsens with weight-bearing.

Early in the disease, the foot retains its normal arch and inversion strength. Tenderness and swelling are noted along the tendon behind the medial malleolus. Resisted inversion or heel raises may elicit pain or weakness. As degeneration progresses, the tendon elongates or tears, leading to collapse of the medial arch (acquired pes planovalgus). The heel drifts into valgus and the "too many toes" sign appears (visible lateral forefoot when viewed from behind). Patients eventually cannot perform a single-leg heel raise on the affected side [4].

Peroneal Tendinopathy [10]

Peroneal tendinopathy involves chronic degeneration or tears of the peroneus brevis and/or longus tendons along the lateral ankle. It often arises in athletes or individuals with a cavovarus foot alignment. Patients typically report posterolateral ankle pain, especially with activities that stress eversion. Examination shows tenderness just behind the lateral malleolus (peroneus brevis course) and possibly pain along the cuboid (peroneus longus). Passive inversion stretches or resisted eversion reproduces discomfort [10]. A forefoot running gait or chronic lateral ankle instability can predispose to these injuries. Tendon subluxation or tears should be suspected if palpation elicits a snapping or if there is a palpable retro malleolar defect.

Retrocalcaneal Bursitis [11]

Retrocalcaneal bursitis (Achilles bursitis) is inflammation of the bursa located between the Achilles tendon and the calcaneus. It typically occurs with insertional Achilles tendinopathy. Patients have posterior heel pain and swelling 1–2 cm above the heel. Dorsiflexion or squeezing the calcaneus against the Achilles exaggerates the pain. A tender, sometimes erythematous swelling may be palpable at the Achilles insertion. Contributing factors include tight calf musculature, overuse, ill-fitting footwear or a prominent Haglund's deformity. Systemic inflammatory arthritides can also predispose to Achilles enthesopathies and bursitis [12].

Flexor Hallucis Longus Tendonitis and Tarsal Tunnel Syndrome [13]

Flexor hallucis longus (FHL) tendonitis ("dancer's tendinitis") causes posterior-medial ankle pain, often in ballet dancers or activities with repetitive toe push-off. Pain is elicited by resisted great-toe flexion or passive forced dorsiflexion of the toe. Tarsal tunnel syndrome is tibial nerve entrapment beneath the flexor retinaculum at the medial ankle. It produces burning, tingling or numbness along the plantar surface of the foot. Exam may reveal a positive Tinel's sign over the tarsal tunnel and sensory deficits in the tibial nerve distribution.

Differentiating Soft Tissue Pathology from Inflammatory Arthropathy and Deformity

It is important to distinguish mechanical tendinopathies from rheumatic disease. Enthesitis (inflammation of tendon/ligament insertions) is characteristic of seronegative spondyloarthropathies [14]. Enthesitis pain tends to be bilateral, with concurrent symptoms (back pain, skin lesions, GI symptoms). In contrast, mechanical tendinopathies are often unilateral or related to overuse, without systemic signs. For example, plantar fasciitis and Achilles tendinosis in an otherwise healthy individual are most often noninflammatory.

Rheumatoid arthritis typically causes symmetric synovitis of the foot joints (MTP, ankle) rather than isolated tendonitis [15]. RA may cause tenosynovitis of foot flexor tendons, but pain is usually joint-centred with morning stiffness. Chronic gout often affects first MTP, not plantar fascia or Achilles [15].

Structural deformities must also be considered. A progressive flatfoot (pes planovalgus) with pain suggests PTTD, whereas fixed deformities may reflect midfoot arthritis. In examining a patient, note arch height, hindfoot alignment (varus/valgus) and the presence of entheseal bone changes on imaging.

Key differences on exam and history: inflammatory enthesitis often has prolonged morning stiffness and systemic features, whereas tendinopathy pain is activity-related. Imaging can help: enthesitis may show bone marrow oedema and enhanced signal at tendon insertions on MRI, while tendinosis shows tendon thickening and degenerative changes. X-rays may reveal enthesophytes (bone spurs) in chronic enthesitis, whereas plantar calcaneal spurs in plantar fasciitis are incidental findings.

Physical Examination [16]

A thorough foot and ankle exam includes inspection, palpation, range of motion and functional testing. Observe the patient standing and walking. Look for arch deformities (pes planus or cavus), hindfoot varus/valgus and gait abnormalities. The "too many toes" sign (forefoot digits visible from behind) suggests flatfoot/PTTD.

Palpation [16]
Systematically palpate tender spots: medial calcaneus (plantar fascia origin), posterior calcaneus (Achilles insertion and bursa), anterior ankle, medial malleolus (tibialis posterior tendon), lateral malleolus (peroneal tendons), base of fifth metatarsal (peroneus brevis) and first metatarsal head. Pain in these sites helps localise pathology.

Resisted Testing [17]
Ask the patient to actively contract tendons against resistance. Pain with resisted plantarflexion suggests Achilles involvement; resisted inversion of the foot (tibialis posterior) or inversion of a plantarflexed foot produces pain in posterior tibial tendinopathy. Resisted foot eversion or plantarflexion reproduces pain in peroneal tendinopathy. Pain with resisted flexion of the great toe indicates FHL tendonitis.

Functional Tests Perform single-leg heel raise: inability or pain on the medial heel during heel raise suggests PTTD [4]. Asking the patient to stand on tiptoes tests Achilles function: inability indicates significant Achilles pathology. The Windlass test (passively dorsiflexing the great toe while the foot is weight-bearing) stretches the plantar fascia; reproduction of heel pain is a positive sign [8].

Neurological Exam Include peripheral pulses and sensory testing. Elicit a Tinel's sign at the tarsal tunnel (percuss posterior to the medial malleolus) if neuropathy is suspected.

Gait Evaluation Observe walking on heels (tests ankle dorsiflexors) and on toes (tests plantar flexors). Note pronation or supination of the foot during stance.

Imaging [18]

Imaging is guided by clinical suspicion. Plain radiographs are indicated in chronic cases (≥6 weeks) or when fracture/deformity is a concern. Heel X-rays may show calcaneal spurs (common in plantar fasciitis) or a Haglund's deformity. Weight-bearing foot films can quantify arch collapse (e.g. decreased calcaneal pitch).

Ultrasound (US) is valuable for soft tissue detail. It can demonstrate tendon thickening, hypoechogenicity, neovascularisation, partial tears and bursitis [19]. Ultrasound is dynamic and can reveal tendon subluxation (peroneal). It is also used to guide corticosteroid or PRP injections for accuracy.

MRI provides detailed visualisation of soft tissues and bone marrow. MRI can detect bone oedema at entheses (suggesting enthesitis), tendon degeneration, partial or full-thickness tears and occult stress injuries. It is useful when diagnosis is unclear or to plan surgery. However, MRI is generally reserved for patients who fail conservative therapy or when complex pathology is suspected.

Management

Conservative Management [20]

For most foot/ankle tendinopathies, non-operative care is first line. This includes *relative rest* and activity modification to offload the affected structure. Ice or cold packs applied after activity can reduce pain. While these are termed "-itis", the conditions are largely degenerative; NSAIDs and paracetamol may provide short-term analgesia but have limited impact on the healing of tendinosis.

Addressing biomechanics is crucial. Stretching exercises are fundamental: patients should perform daily calf (gastrocnemius and soleus) and plantar fascia stretches. Strengthening the foot and ankle musculature is also important. Eccentric loading programmes are recommended for Achilles and PTTD, as they have been shown to improve pain and function. For plantar fasciitis, exercises that stretch and load the fascia (standing calf stretches, towel stretches) are advised. Night splints that dorsiflex the foot may help some patients by keeping the plantar fascia lengthened during sleep.

Orthotic support can correct foot alignment. Over-the-counter or custom shoe inserts with medial arch support are often helpful in plantar fasciitis and PTTD. A heel lift or cushion can offload the Achilles insertion. For peroneal tendinopathy, a slight lateral heel wedge may reduce strain. Appropriate footwear (supportive shoes, shock-absorbing soles) is emphasised.

Physiotherapy can incorporate soft tissue mobilisation, taping or bracing and modality treatments. Immobilisation (walking boot or CAM boot) for several weeks may be used for severe acute flares or refractory cases, especially in PTTD or acute ruptures.

Injections and Advanced Therapies [21]

If conservative measures fail, corticosteroid injections under ultrasound guidance can be considered for bursitis or peritendinous inflammation. Steroids should be injected adjacent to (not into) the tendon itself to avoid rupture. The benefit is usually short-term pain relief. Limit steroid injections to a single dose (or at most two) per site due to risk of tendon weakening. Overall, corticosteroid injection around the plantar fascia or Achilles region should be used cautiously because of risks including fascia rupture, fat pad atrophy and tendon weakening; intratendinous injection should be avoided.

Adjunct therapies include platelet-rich plasma (PRP) and extracorporeal shock wave therapy (ESWT). Evidence is mixed, but these may be offered for chronic, refractory tendinosis. For example, shockwave has shown benefit in chronic plantar fasciitis and Achilles tendinosis [22]. PRP injections (often into the tendon sheath or areas of tendon tears) are also used to promote healing, often combined with exercise rehab. These should not replace core conservative treatment.

Surgical intervention is reserved for recalcitrant cases. Indications include tendon rupture, intractable pain despite ≥3–6 months of therapy or progressive deformity. Examples are partial tendon debridement and exostectomy for insertional Achilles tendinopathy, plantar fascia release (open or endoscopic) for unremitting plantar fasciitis and tendon repair and osteotomies for advanced PTTD. Rheumatologists should refer to orthopaedic surgery when structural reconstruction or release procedures are needed or when inflammatory arthritis is suspected (e.g. refractory enthesitis in SpA).

Prognosis and Prevention

Prognosis is generally favourable with appropriate treatment, but recovery can be slow. About 70–80% of plantar fasciitis patients improve within 9–12 months of conservative therapy [8]. Similarly, most Achilles and PTT tendinopathies respond to 3–6 months of exercise and therapy, although symptoms can recur if biomechanics remain uncorrected. A small percentage (around 5–10%) of plantar fasciitis cases may eventually require surgical release [23].

Preventive strategies include graduated training (avoid sudden increases in activity), regular calf and plantar fascia stretching and proper footwear selection. Eccentric strengthening exercises can be begun early in high-risk patients. Measures such as weight management and avoiding prolonged barefoot walking on hard surfaces can reduce stress on the foot. Patients should be counselled on these preventive approaches to minimise recurrence.

Key Learning Points

- Foot and ankle tendon disorders are commonly degenerative (tendinosis or enthesopathy) rather than inflammatory. Diagnosis relies on clinical history and exam.
- Achilles tendinopathy can be mid-portion or insertional; exam shows tendon tenderness and pain with resisted plantarflexion.
- Plantar fasciitis presents with stabbing heel pain on first steps (windlass test can reproduce pain). Risk factors include foot arch abnormalities and tight calves.
- Posterior tibial tendinopathy (PTTD) often leads to a flexible flatfoot; look for medial hindfoot pain and inability to do single-leg heel raises.
- Peroneal tendinopathy causes lateral ankle pain; exam reveals tenderness behind the lateral malleolus and pain with eversion stress.
- Differentiate these from inflammatory conditions: bilateral enthesitis in spondyloarthritis often accompanies systemic features. RA usually affects joints symmetrically, not isolated entheses.
- Physical exam: palpate specific tendons/entheses; perform functional tests (heel raises, gait). Utilise imaging selectively: X-ray for bone changes and US or MRI for soft tissue pathology.

- Management is primarily conservative: physiotherapy with stretching and eccentric exercises, orthoses, NSAIDs (for pain relief) and patient education.
- Ultrasound-guided injections (steroids, PRP) and shockwave therapy are options for refractory cases.
- Refer if symptoms remain refractory despite an adequate structured rehabilitation period, typically 6–12 months, or earlier if rupture, progressive deformity, neurological compromise or diagnostic uncertainty is present.
- Emphasise biomechanical correction and prevention: proper shoes, gradual training increases and weight control improve outcomes.

References

1. Gomes TM, Oliva XM, Viridiana Sanchez E, Soares S, Diaz T. Anatomy of the ankle and subtalar joint ligaments: what we do not know about it? Foot Ankle Clin [Internet]. 2023;28(2):201–16. Available from: http://www.ncbi.nlm.nih.gov/pubmed/37137619.
2. Medina Pabón MA, Naqvi U. Achilles Tendinopathy [Internet]. StatPearls. 2023. Available from: https://www.ncbi.nlm.nih.gov/books/NBK538149/.
3. Stecco C, Corradin M, Macchi V, Morra A, Porzionato A, Biz C, et al. Plantar fascia anatomy and its relationship with Achilles tendon and paratenon. J Anat [Internet]. 2013;223(6):665–76. Available from: http://www.ncbi.nlm.nih.gov/pubmed/24028383.
4. Knapp PW, Constant D. Posterior Tibial Tendon Dysfunction [Internet]. StatPearls. 2026. Available from: http://www.ncbi.nlm.nih.gov/pubmed/30271611.
5. Chan CW, Rudins A. Foot biomechanics during walking and running. Mayo Clin Proc [Internet]. 1994;69(5):448–61. Available from: http://www.ncbi.nlm.nih.gov/pubmed/8170197.
6. Chimenti RL, Cychosz CC, Hall MM, Phisitkul P. Current concepts review update: insertional Achilles tendinopathy. Foot ankle Int [Internet]. 2017;38(10):1160–9. Available from: http://www.ncbi.nlm.nih.gov/pubmed/28789557.
7. Bolon B. Mini-review: toxic tendinopathy. Toxicol Pathol [Internet]. 2017;45(7):834–7. Available from: http://www.ncbi.nlm.nih.gov/pubmed/28553748.
8. Buchanan BK, Sina RE, Kushner D. Plantar Fasciitis [Internet]. StatPearls. 2026. Available from: http://www.ncbi.nlm.nih.gov/pubmed/37025731.
9. Trojian T, Tucker AK. Plantar Fasciitis. Am Fam Physician [Internet]. 2019;99(12):744–50. Available from: http://www.ncbi.nlm.nih.gov/pubmed/31194492.
10. Walt J, Massey P. Peroneal Tendon Syndromes [Internet]. StatPearls. 2023. Available from: https://www.ncbi.nlm.nih.gov/books/NBK544354/.
11. Pękala PA, Henry BM, Pękala JR, Piska K, Tomaszewski KA. The Achilles tendon and the retrocalcaneal bursa: an anatomical and radiological study. Bone Joint Res [Internet]. 2017;6(7):446–51. Available from: http://www.ncbi.nlm.nih.gov/pubmed/28765268.
12. Suzuki T, Hidaka Y, Seri Y. Retrocalcaneal bursitis precedes or accompanies Achilles tendon enthesitis in the early phase of rheumatoid arthritis. Clin Med Insights Arthritis Musculoskelet Disord [Internet]. 2018;11:1179544118781094. Available from: http://www.ncbi.nlm.nih.gov/pubmed/29899668.
13. Kiel J, Kaiser K. Tarsal Tunnel Syndrome [Internet]. StatPearls. 2024. Available from: https://www.ncbi.nlm.nih.gov/books/NBK513273/.
14. Sudoł-Szopińska I, Kwiatkowska B, Prochorec-Sobieszek M, Maśliński W. Enthesopathies and enthesitis. Part 1. etiopathogenesis. J Ultrason [Internet]. 2015;15(60):72–84. Available from: http://www.ncbi.nlm.nih.gov/pubmed/26674568

15. Giraudo C, Fichera G, Ganguly S, Arumugam M, Cecchin D, Rennie WJ. Ankle and foot: focus on inflammatory disease. Semin Musculoskelet Radiol [Internet]. 2023;27(3):327–36. Available from: http://www.ncbi.nlm.nih.gov/pubmed/37230132.
16. Alazzawi S, Sukeik M, King D, Vemulapalli K. Foot and ankle history and clinical examination: a guide to everyday practice. World J Orthop [Internet]. 2017;8(1):21–9. Available from: http://www.ncbi.nlm.nih.gov/pubmed/28144575.
17. Young CC, Niedfeldt MW, Morris GA, Eerkes KJ. Clinical examination of the foot and ankle. Prim Care [Internet]. 2005;32(1):105–32. Available from: http://www.ncbi.nlm.nih.gov/pubmed/15831315.
18. Papineni VRK, Mariathas M, Sidhu SS, Chari B. Imaging modalities for non-acute pathologies of the foot and ankle. J Clin Orthop trauma [Internet]. 2024;48:102329. Available from: http://www.ncbi.nlm.nih.gov/pubmed/38299021.
19. Elsaman AM, Mostafa ES, Radwan AR. Ankle evaluation in active rheumatoid arthritis by ultrasound: a cross-sectional study. Ultrasound Med Biol [Internet]. 2017;43(12):2806–13. Available from: https://linkinghub.elsevier.com/retrieve/pii/S0301562917312899.
20. Hong CC, Pearce CJ, Ballal MS, Calder JDF. Management of sports injuries of the foot and ankle: an update. Bone Joint J [Internet]. 2016;98-B(10):1299–311. Available from: http://www.ncbi.nlm.nih.gov/pubmed/27694582.
21. de Cesar NC, da Fonseca LF, Simeone Nascimento F, O'Daley AE, Tan EW, Dein EJ, et al. ☆Diagnostic and therapeutic injections of the foot and ankle-an overview. Foot Ankle Surg [Internet]. 2018;24(2):99–106. Available from: http://www.ncbi.nlm.nih.gov/pubmed/29409219.
22. Wilson M, Stacy J. Shock wave therapy for Achilles tendinopathy. Curr Rev Musculoskelet Med [Internet]. 2010;4(1):6–10. Available from: http://www.ncbi.nlm.nih.gov/pubmed/21475558.
23. Sahu RL. Percutaneous planter fasciitis release under local anesthesia: a prospective study. Chinese J Traumatol = Zhonghua chuang shang za zhi [Internet]. 2017;20(2):87–9. Available from: http://www.ncbi.nlm.nih.gov/pubmed/28336421.

Generalised Soft Tissue Pain and Fibromyalgia

11

Abstract

Fibromyalgia is a chronic pain syndrome characterised by widespread musculoskeletal pain, fatigue, non-restorative sleep and cognitive disturbance. It exemplifies generalised soft tissue pain without a primary inflammatory or structural lesion. This chapter reviews definitions and diagnostic criteria for fibromyalgia and related entities such as myofascial pain syndrome and hypermobility-associated pain. Clinical features are discussed alongside diagnostic challenges, including the overlap of fibromyalgia with chronic fatigue syndrome and other functional somatic syndromes. Management is multifaceted: patient education, exercise and cognitive behavioural therapy (CBT) form the cornerstone, with judicious use of pharmacotherapy for symptom relief. Special considerations in fibromyalgia care—such as stigma, validation and effective doctor-patient communication—are highlighted. The role of the rheumatologist in diagnosis and co-management is explored, including when to refer patients for specialist care. Key learning points are summarised to reinforce an evidence-based, patient-centred approach to generalised soft tissue pain and fibromyalgia.

Case Vignette

Case A 45-year-old woman presents with a 5-year history of diffuse musculoskeletal pain. Her pain began insidiously and has gradually worsened; it is present "all over" but especially in the neck, shoulders and lower back. She reports unrelenting fatigue and unrefreshing sleep, often waking up feeling as tired as the night before. She has difficulty concentrating at work and notes frequent headaches and irritable bowel syndrome symptoms. Over the years, she has seen multiple physicians and underwent numerous tests (including rheumatological blood tests, MRI scans and thyroid evaluations), all of which were unrevealing. One doctor told her "nothing is wrong" and suggested stress as the cause, leaving her feeling frustrated and

© The Author(s), under exclusive license to Springer Nature Switzerland AG 2026
R. Amarnani, *Soft Tissue and Musculoskeletal Medicine in Rheumatology*,
https://doi.org/10.1007/978-3-032-29441-8_11

stigmatised. On examination, there is no synovitis or overt joint pathology, but she has tenderness in many soft tissue sites, including classic tender points in trapezius, elbows and hips. The patient is tearful, expressing relief that "finally someone believes my pain is real".

Discussion This case highlights a classic presentation of fibromyalgia, including widespread pain, fatigue and normal investigative results. It underscores the importance of compassionate listening and the challenges patients face in obtaining a diagnosis. A focused management plan addressing education, exercise and supportive therapies would be the next step.

Definitions and Diagnostic Criteria

Fibromyalgia Fibromyalgia (FM) is a chronic, generalised pain syndrome defined by widespread musculoskeletal pain accompanied by fatigue, sleep disturbances, cognitive dysfunction and a constellation of other somatic symptoms [1]. It is classified as a central sensitisation syndrome, meaning the nervous system is in a heightened state of sensitivity and reactivity, leading to pain amplification without a primary inflammatory or structural lesion explaining the full symptom burden. FM is common, with prevalence estimates ranging from around 2–4% of the general population, predominantly affecting women in midlife [2]. Patients often describe pain as "all over" or migratory, and they experience stiffness, particularly in the morning or after inactivity, though objective joint swelling is absent. Fatigue in fibromyalgia can be profound, and patients commonly report light, unrefreshing sleep [3].

Myofascial Pain Syndrome
Myofascial pain syndrome (MPS) is a regional pain condition caused by myofascial trigger points within muscles [4]. Unlike fibromyalgia, which is generalised, MPS is usually localised to one or a few regions (e.g. neck-shoulder or low back pain due to trigger points in those muscles). A trigger point is defined as a hyperirritable spot in a taut band of skeletal muscle fascia that is painful on compression and can evoke characteristic referred pain, tenderness and even autonomic phenomena. On examination, clinicians can often feel a firm, ropy band in the muscle and find a focal tender nodule—pressure on this point reproduces the patient's typical pain (which may radiate in a specific pattern). For example, a trigger point in the upper trapezius might refer pain upward into the head (tension headache) or down the arm. Diagnostic criteria for myofascial trigger points have varied, but a general consensus is that the essential findings include a palpable taut band in the muscle, a hyperirritable tender spot within that band and referred pain elicited by stimulating that spot [4]. Often there may be a local twitch response (a brief muscle contraction) when snapping the band and limited range of motion or muscle weakness due to pain. MPS is a common contributor to musculoskeletal pain. For instance, many cases of chronic neck or back pain have a myofascial component. It may occur on

its own or in conjunction with other conditions (including fibromyalgia—some fibromyalgia patients also have active myofascial trigger points). Differentiating MPS from fibromyalgia is important: MPS is typically regional rather than widespread, and trigger point injections or other local therapies can be particularly effective for MPS, whereas fibromyalgia requires more global management.

Hypermobility-Related Pain Generalised joint hypermobility refers to increased range of motion in multiple joints beyond normal limits. While many people with hypermobility are asymptomatic (e.g. young individuals or dancers/gymnasts), a subset experience chronic pain due to repetitive microtrauma, joint instability and strain on soft tissues [5]. When hypermobility is accompanied by chronic musculoskeletal pain and other symptoms in the absence of another systemic rheumatic disease, it is often termed joint hypermobility syndrome (JHS) or, as per newer classification, part of the hypermobility spectrum disorders [6]. The most notable heritable disorder of connective tissue in this realm is hypermobile Ehlers-Danlos syndrome (hEDS), diagnosed by specific criteria (which include generalised hypermobility, plus skin/soft tissue findings and familial history). Patients with hypermobility-related pain often present with joint pain that fluctuates, frequent sprains or injuries and a history of being "double-jointed".

On exam they have a high Beighton score (a nine-point scale assessing flexibility of knees, elbows, thumbs, little fingers and spine). For instance, they can often bend forward and place palms on the floor, hyperextend elbows or knees beyond 10°, etc. Over time, repeated joint subluxations or microinjuries can lead to chronic pain that may resemble fibromyalgia in its diffuseness. Indeed, there is considerable overlap between hypermobility syndromes and fibromyalgia: recent data suggest that a large proportion of patients with hypermobile EDS or hypermobility spectrum disorders also meet criteria for fibromyalgia and vice versa [6]. Both conditions share features like pain, fatigue and autonomic symptoms. The mechanism may involve chronic pain input from unstable joints leading to central sensitisation [7]. Recognising hypermobility is important because management includes stabilising joints (through targeted exercises, bracing, activity modification) in addition to the general fibromyalgia strategies. Hypermobility-related pain syndromes highlight the importance of a thorough history and exam: what might initially be labelled as "widespread pain" could in some cases be pain stemming from multiple hypermobile joints and soft tissue injuries.

In summary, fibromyalgia, myofascial pain syndrome and hypermobility-related pain are distinct yet sometimes overlapping entities within the spectrum of generalised soft tissue pain. Fibromyalgia is a widespread pain condition defined by central sensitisation and broad symptomatology; myofascial pain is a regional pain disorder of trigger points; and hypermobility-related pain arises from connective tissue laxity and joint instability. A patient can have one or a combination of these—for example, a person with hypermobility might develop secondary myofascial trigger points, or a fibromyalgia patient might also have active trigger areas. A careful evaluation is required to identify these components, as it guides tailored management.

Clinical Features and Diagnostic Challenges

Clinical Features of Fibromyalgia Patients with fibromyalgia typically report chronic, diffuse pain that has been present for many months or years. The pain is often described as a deep ache but can also have stabbing, burning or throbbing qualities. It may begin in one region (such as the neck and shoulders) and generalise over time [1]. Pain is usually worse with physical or emotional stress, poor sleep or inactivity, and some patients note weather changes can affect symptoms. Besides pain, fatigue is a hallmark—often severe enough to impair daily activities and not proportional to exertion. Patients struggle with unrefreshing sleep; even with adequate hours, they wake feeling tired. This is often due to sleep fragmentation (possibly from alpha-wave intrusions during deep sleep). Cognitive difficulties are another key feature—patients may have trouble with memory, attention and word finding, which they find distressing especially if it affects work or multitasking. Mood disturbances are common: anxiety and depression occur in a substantial subset (roughly 30–50% or more) of fibromyalgia patients [2], and even in those without formal psychiatric diagnoses, chronic pain often leads to frustration, worry or low mood. A variety of somatic symptoms often cooccur [8]: tension or migraine headaches, irritable bowel syndrome (IBS) causing abdominal pain and bloating, irritable bladder or interstitial cystitis (urinary frequency/pain), temporomandibular joint pain, premenstrual syndrome, restless legs syndrome, paraesthesias (numbness or tingling in extremities) and subjective swelling of hands or feet. On examination, fibromyalgia patients usually appear well with no joint inflammation or muscle weakness. Neurological exam is grossly normal aside from tenderness. Widespread tender points or generalised hyperalgesia can be elicited—gentle pressure on soft tissue spots (trapezius, medial knees, lateral elbows, etc.) reproduces pain.

Fibromyalgia has no verified or specific laboratory or imaging markers [9]. Routine tests (e.g. inflammatory markers, thyroid function, muscle enzymes) are typically normal. This lack of objective findings is a core challenge and partly why fibromyalgia was historically a diagnosis of exclusion. However, current thinking is that fibromyalgia can be diagnosed clinically if the pattern fits and other diseases are reasonably ruled out. In practice, diagnostic work-up is usually aimed at excluding mimicking conditions: for example, thyroid disease (hypothyroidism can cause fatigue and myalgias), vitamin D deficiency, anaemia or occult inflammatory diseases. If history or exam suggests, one might check RF, anti-CCP, ANA or other autoimmune tests should be reserved for patients with features suggestive of inflammatory arthritis or connective tissue disease, but widespread pain with normal exam and blood tests is most often fibromyalgia.

Clinical Features of Myofascial Pain Syndrome [4] Myofascial pain presents with regional pain syndromes. The pain is often dull or aching but can flare into sharper pain on certain movements or stress. It commonly radiates in specific patterns; patients may not be aware of the radiation until the clinician palpates a trigger point that reproduces pain distant from the pressure site. Stiffness and a feeling of knotted muscles are common. Unlike fibromyalgia, myofascial pain may have a precipitating factor such as a localised muscle injury, poor posture or repetitive strain. Patients might say "I have a knot in my shoulder" or report a tight band that when pressed "good hurt" and relieves pain temporarily. On exam, the hallmark is finding the taut band and trigger point. Applying pressure causes local tenderness, a jump or wince response and referred pain. There may be a reduced range of motion in the affected muscle group (e.g. decreased cervical rotation due to neck muscle trigger points). No systemic features (fever, weight loss) are present. Laboratory tests are normal. The diagnosis is clinical; one challenge is that it requires an experienced examiner to detect trigger points reliably, and there is some examiner variability. There is no routinely used imaging test that reliably confirms trigger points in standard clinical practice, though techniques like ultrasound or MRI elastography are being researched to visualise the palpable nodules. The absence of a definitive test means myofascial pain can be underdiagnosed or misdiagnosed as other pain syndromes. Conversely, overdiagnosis can occur if every regional pain is labelled "myofascial" without careful exam confirmation.

Clinical Features of Hypermobility-Related Pain Patients with hypermobility spectrum disorders or hEDS often present with pain in multiple joints, frequently worsening towards evening or after physical activity. They might describe joints that easily "pop" or partially dislocate. For example, they may wake up with shoulder pain from a minor subluxation during sleep or sprain their ankles frequently when walking on uneven ground. Back pain is common due to ligamentous laxity in the spine and pelvis. They often have a history of being very flexible in youth (e.g. doing splits, contortionist tricks) and may have other signs like stretchy skin, easy bruising or autonomic symptoms (in hEDS, conditions like POTS—postural tachycardia—are reported). Fatigue can be present, partly from the effort of stabilising joints. On exam, the key feature is generalised hypermobility: a Beighton score of ≥5/9 is commonly used in adults up to age 50 (e.g. passive dorsiflexion of little finger >90°, thumb touching forearm, elbows/knees hyperextending >10°, forward bending palms to floor) is indicative [10]. Joints may demonstrate excessive range with pain at end range. There may be tenderness at sites of chronic strain (e.g. medial knee from collateral ligament strain, low back from ligamentous support issues). Muscle tone might be somewhat increased as muscles try to compensate for lax ligaments. Similar to fibromyalgia, standard blood tests are normal. The diagnosis of hypermobility syndrome or hEDS is made by clinical criteria; genetic testing exists for most subtypes of Ehlers-Danlos but not for the hypermobile type. A diagnostic challenge is that hypermobility-related pain can be mistaken for fibromyalgia (both involve multisite pain and fatigue). Indeed, they can overlap. One clue is the nature of the pain—in hypermobility, pain often centres around joints and may improve with joint bracing or avoidance of extreme movements, whereas fibromyalgia pain is more widespread in muscles and soft tissues and less activity-specific. Another clue is the exam: hypermobile patients demonstrably have lax joints, whereas fibromyalgia patients primarily have tenderness. It is possible for a patient to satisfy criteria for both hEDS and fibromyalgia; in such cases, both diagnoses should be recognised, as management will need to address both central pain and peripheral joint stability.

Diagnostic Challenges Diagnosing fibromyalgia and related soft tissue pain syndromes can be challenging for several reasons:

- *Lack of objective markers:* Fibromyalgia does not have a clear biomarker or imaging finding. Its lab tests are normal, and even muscle biopsies show nonspecific changes at best. This can make some clinicians (and patients) uneasy with the diagnosis, feeling that "something must have been missed". Myofascial pain and hypermobility also lack easy objective tests (aside from the Beighton exam for hypermobility, which itself requires examiner familiarity). The clinician must rely on patient history and physical exam. This requires time and careful attention, which is not always provided in busy practice settings.
- *Overlap with other conditions:* Fibromyalgia symptoms overlap with many other diagnoses. For example, hypothyroidism, vitamin D deficiency, anaemia or sleep apnoea can cause fatigue and generalised aches [11]. Rheumatoid arthritis or SLE can initially present with diffuse pain and fatigue (even before obvious swelling or lab abnormalities appear), leading to potential confusion. Conversely, once a patient is labelled with fibromyalgia, there is a risk that new symptoms might be prematurely attributed to fibro when in fact another condition (like an autoimmune flare or degenerative arthritis) has developed. Clinicians must maintain an open mind and periodically reassess for coexisting disorders.
- *Multiple syndromes coexisting:* It is not uncommon for a patient to meet criteria for several syndromes simultaneously, for example, fibromyalgia *and* chronic fatigue syndrome, or fibromyalgia *and* hypermobility syndrome, etc. This can complicate diagnostic labelling and management, as such patients have a high symptom burden. The concept of central sensitivity syndromes (CSS) was proposed to group these together, including fibromyalgia, irritable bowel, tension headache, temporomandibular disorder, chronic fatigue syndrome and others that have overlapping features. Recognising the overlap can help validate patients (their myriad symptoms are part of an understood pattern) but also poses a challenge in coordinating care across specialties.
- *Stigma and physician attitudes* [12]: A significant challenge is that some healthcare providers have historically been sceptical about fibromyalgia. Patients often report feeling that their previous doctors did not "believe" in the illness. Unfortunately, remnants of this stigma persist. This gap underscores that many patients see multiple providers before getting a proper diagnosis. The inconsistency in physician knowledge and acceptance means patients may receive conflicting messages, adding to their frustration and delaying effective care.
- *Psychological factors:* Conditions like fibromyalgia exist at a nexus of physical and psychological domains. While fibromyalgia is *not* "all in the head," stress and emotional state can modulate symptoms due to the mind-body connection. Patients under high stress or with unresolved trauma (which is not uncommon in

fibromyalgia histories) might have intensified pain perception. This interplay can muddle the diagnostic process, for example, distinguishing fibromyalgia from somatic symptom disorder or depression-related aches. A careful, empathetic approach is needed to untangle these factors without invalidating the patient's physical suffering.

In confronting these diagnostic challenges, a thorough but judicious approach is key. The evaluation of chronic widespread pain should include a detailed history (covering pain characteristics, triggers, associated symptoms, stressors, sleep quality) and a comprehensive physical exam (looking for tender points, trigger points, hypermobility, muscle spasm, true joint swelling, neurologic deficits, skin changes, etc.). Initial laboratory tests often include a complete blood count, ESR/CRP (inflammatory markers), TSH, perhaps creatine kinase and age-appropriate screenings (like calcium/vitamin D and others if indicated)—primarily to exclude other diagnoses. In patients with red flag signs or atypical features, further tests or referrals are warranted (e.g. if significant objective joint swelling, then autoimmune serologies or referral to rheumatology; if profound fatigue with orthostatic symptoms, consider testing for orthostatic intolerance; etc.). Often, by the time fibromyalgia is diagnosed, patients have already had extensive testing. The challenge then becomes avoiding overinvestigation—once fibromyalgia is established, repetitive imaging or labs in search of a nonexistent structural cause can be harmful and wasteful. At the same time, clinicians must remain vigilant to any new developments that suggest an alternate or additional diagnosis. Striking this balance is an art of medical practice.

Overlaps with Chronic Fatigue Syndrome and Functional Syndromes

Fibromyalgia does not exist in isolation; it can often overlap with other chronic overlapping conditions, including ME/CFS, IBS, migraine and temporomandibular disorder. Chronic fatigue syndrome (CFS), also known as myalgic encephalomyelitis (ME/CFS), is one such condition [13]. Both fibromyalgia and CFS feature severe fatigue, unrefreshing sleep and cognitive issues. In CFS, fatigue (especially *postexertional malaise*, the hallmark where even minor physical or mental exertion can lead to a crash of worsening symptoms) is the predominant complaint, whereas in fibromyalgia, pain is predominant—but many patients fulfil criteria for both. Estimates vary, but a considerable proportion of fibromyalgia patients (perhaps 20–70%) also meet criteria for CFS and vice versa [14]. Clinically, when both are present, the patient's suffering is high—they experience both significant pain and profound exhaustion. Management principles for fibromyalgia and CFS overlap in areas of graded exercise (with careful pacing), cognitive therapies and addressing sleep, though CFS typically requires even more cautious pacing due to postexertional worsening.

Other functional somatic syndromes frequently cooccur, forming a cluster of interrelated conditions [8]:

- *Irritable bowel syndrome (IBS):* Characterised by chronic abdominal pain with altered bowel habits, IBS is reported by a large subset of fibromyalgia patients. The visceral hypersensitivity in IBS (e.g. bloating, pain with normal gut distension) parallels the central pain amplification in fibromyalgia. Both conditions improve with centrally-acting therapies like low-dose antidepressants, suggesting shared pathophysiology.
- *Tension headaches/migraines:* Chronic headaches, particularly tension-type headaches (dull, band-like pain) and migraine headaches, are more common in fibromyalgia. Muscle tension in the neck/upper back (myofascial trigger points) can trigger headaches, and central sensitisation can amplify headache pain. Many fibromyalgia patients describe frequent headaches that significantly impact quality of life.
- *Temporomandibular disorder (TMD):* This presents as jaw pain, chewing difficulty and jaw joint clicking. It is essentially myofascial pain in the masticatory muscles and often coexists with fibromyalgia. Patients with fibromyalgia have a higher prevalence of TMD than the general population.
- *Restless legs syndrome (RLS):* An uncomfortable sensation in the legs at rest, relieved by movement, leading to insomnia—RLS is more common in fibromyalgia patients, contributing to their sleep disruption.
- *Interstitial cystitis/painful bladder syndrome:* Chronic bladder pain and urinary frequency can occur; many fibromyalgia patients report some urological symptoms, and studies show a higher incidence of interstitial cystitis in this group than expected.
- *Depression and anxiety disorders:* As mentioned, there is overlap not just in comorbidity but also in symptom expression. For example, panic attacks or generalised anxiety may heighten pain perception and muscle tension, while depression can magnify fatigue and sleep problems. In some patients, it is challenging to discern where one syndrome ends and another begins (e.g. is it fibromyalgia with secondary depression, or depression with somatic symptoms? Often it is both).

For the clinician, recognising these overlaps is important for several reasons:

- It prompts a holistic assessment. A fibromyalgia patient might also need evaluation for IBS if they have GI complaints, or a patient with CFS symptoms should be asked about pain and potentially meet fibromyalgia criteria.
- It supports multidisciplinary management. For instance, such a patient may benefit from a pain specialist, a gastroenterologist and a psychologist working in concert.
- It aids patient education. Patients often feel relieved to know that their seemingly disparate symptoms (bowel problems, headaches, pain, fatigue) may all be connected.

- It requires prioritisation of treatments that address multiple symptoms. Exercise therapy, for example, can improve fibromyalgia pain, reduce fatigue, improve IBS constipation and help mood—a broad-spectrum intervention. Similarly, medications like duloxetine can potentially help pain, headaches and anxiety/depression together.

However, overlapping syndromes also mean that patients can end up seeing many specialists who each focus on one organ system, sometimes resulting in polypharmacy and fragmented care. It falls often to rheumatologists or primary care physicians to play the role of integrator to avoid this fragmentation.

In summary, fibromyalgia overlaps extensively with chronic fatigue syndrome and other functional somatic syndromes, sharing mechanisms of central sensitisation. These overlaps can complicate diagnosis and management but, when recognised, also offer an opportunity for a unified, biopsychosocial treatment strategy. The suffering of patients with multiple syndromes is very real and often severe—validating this and avoiding unnecessary interventions (e.g. repeated endoscopies for IBS or endless imaging for headaches once serious pathology is excluded) is a key aspect of care. The focus should shift from exhaustive investigation to comprehensive management addressing the patient's global well-being.

Management Strategies

Management of fibromyalgia and generalised soft tissue pain conditions requires a multimodal approach [15]. Given the complex interplay of physical, psychological and social factors, no single treatment is a magic bullet. Instead, combining patient education, non-pharmacologic therapies (like exercise and CBT) and targeted pharmacotherapy yields the best outcomes. The emphasis is on improving function and quality of life rather than eliminating pain completely (an unrealistic goal in most chronic pain syndromes). Below we outline the main strategies:

Patient Education and Reassurance [16]

Education is the *foundation* of fibromyalgia management. Patients often come to the rheumatologist after months or years of confusion and worry, sometimes believing they have a serious undiagnosed disease. Taking time to explain the diagnosis and its implications is therapeutic in itself. Key points to communicate include the following:

- *Validation:* Explain that fibromyalgia is a real, recognised medical condition—not "in your head". It has neurochemical and physiological underpinnings (such as central sensitisation, altered pain signalling and dysautonomia).
- *Benign but impactful nature:* Fibromyalgia (and related soft tissue pain syndromes) are chronic but *not degenerative or deforming*. Unlike rheumatoid

arthritis or lupus, fibromyalgia does not cause joint or organ damage and does not shorten lifespan. This is important for reassurance: "Although your pain is severe, we can say with confidence it is not due to progressive structural damage in your joints or muscles". However, also acknowledge it is *very impactful* on life quality—the goal is to improve day-to-day function despite the chronic nature.

- *Central sensitisation concept:* Using analogies can help. For example, describe pain processing as an amplifier system—in fibromyalgia the volume knob is turned up too high in the nervous system. Even normal signals (like gentle pressure or muscle use) are perceived as pain. This is why tests are normal—it is not a problem detectable in the muscles or joints themselves but in how the body perceives pain. This analogy can help patients (and their family members) understand that lack of findings does not mean lack of pain; it is pain due to a sensitised nervous system.
- *Role of stress and emotions:* Gently discuss how stress, poor sleep or emotional strain can exacerbate symptoms. This is not to say stress *causes* fibromyalgia but that the mind-body connection influences it. Emphasise that managing stress and mood (through techniques like mindfulness or therapy) can translate to less pain—giving the patient a sense of agency.
- *Expectations:* Set realistic goals. For instance, rather than "cure" (which might set them up for disappointment), focus on improving function—for example, being able to walk 30 minutes, or have the energy to do part-time work or enjoy hobbies again. Pain intensity may gradually abate with the right approach, but there will be good and bad days. Explain flares (periods of worse symptoms often triggered by overexertion or illness) and how to manage them. If the patient knows flares can happen and do not indicate new injury, it reduces panic and catastrophising when they occur.
- *Avoiding repeated unhelpful investigations:* Compassionately explain that repeated consultations and investigations, looking for a hidden cause, can become counterproductive once fibromyalgia is established. Tests should be done to rule out other diseases at the start, but after that, the focus should pivot to symptom management. More scans or specialist referrals for every symptom often end up causing frustration or even iatrogenic harm. Encourage the patient to stick with a consistent management plan rather than bouncing around seeking an elusive cure. This often entails building a strong therapeutic alliance: the patient needs to trust that *you* (and your team) will work with them over time to improve their condition.

Educational resources, such as pamphlets or reputable websites (e.g. patient-oriented summaries from rheumatology associations), can reinforce what is discussed. Some patients benefit from support groups or online forums to know they are not alone—though one must caution them to use these positively and be wary of misinformation. Overall, informed patients who understand their condition tend to cope better and are more likely to engage in active management strategies like exercise or therapy.

Exercise and Physical Activity

Exercise is the cornerstone of fibromyalgia therapy and indeed for most chronic musculoskeletal pain syndromes. In fibromyalgia, exercise has the strongest evidence of benefit among all therapies, with consistent findings that regular physical activity improves pain, fatigue and quality of life [17]. Because patients are often deconditioned and apprehensive (they fear activity will worsen pain), the approach to exercise must be gentle, gradual and encouraging.

The types of exercise found beneficial include the following:

- *Aerobic exercise:* Activities such as brisk walking, low-impact aerobics, cycling or aquatic exercise (swimming or water aerobics) are effective. Aerobic conditioning improves muscle endurance and cardiovascular fitness and has analgesic effects via endorphin release and improved blood flow. Even moderate aerobic exercise has been shown to reduce fibromyalgia pain and stiffness and improve sleep and mood [17]. Ideally, patients should build up to ~30 minutes of moderate-intensity aerobic activity on most days of the week (e.g. five days), as tolerated. "Moderate intensity" can be defined as a level that slightly raises heart rate and breathing but still allows conversation (often around 50–70% of age-predicted maximum heart rate). For many fibromyalgia patients, however, the initial target might be much lower—say, 5–10 minutes of walking or gentle cycling, with rest as needed. Over time, the duration can be extended by a few minutes each week. Some patients may start with exercise in a warm water pool, which reduces impact and relaxes muscles (hydrotherapy has the added benefit of warmth and buoyancy, which many fibromyalgia patients find soothing). Importantly, studies show *any* aerobic exercise is better than none, and there is not clear evidence that one form (land vs water or walking vs cycling) is superior [17]—the best exercise is the one the patient will actually do consistently.
- *Strength training:* Resistance exercise (using light weights, resistance bands or bodyweight exercises) helps improve muscle tone, support joints and can reduce pain in the long run by improving physical stability. Strength training was once thought potentially too intense for fibromyalgia, but research indicates it is beneficial when carefully supervised and scaled to the individual. EULAR guidelines note that both aerobic and strengthening exercises are effective [17]. A typical plan might involve two sessions per week of light resistance training focusing on major muscle groups.
- *Flexibility and stretching:* Stretching exercises (e.g. gentle yoga, tai chi, Pilates-based stretching) improve range of motion and may alleviate the feeling of muscle tightness. Many fibromyalgia patients feel "stiff" and benefit from daily stretching of key muscle groups (neck, shoulders, low back, hips, legs). This can also reduce the risk of exercise-related injury and serves as a good warm-up or cool-down around aerobic activity. Mind-body exercises like yoga and tai chi deserve special mention: they combine stretching, gentle strengthening, balance and relaxation techniques. Trials of tai chi and yoga in fibromyalgia have shown improvements in pain and function, comparable in effect size to aerobic exercise

[18]. These activities also encourage body awareness and stress reduction through controlled breathing, which can help break the pain-anxiety cycle.
- *Balance and core stability:* In hypermobility patients or those with deconditioning, including exercises for core strengthening and balance (proprioception) can prevent falls and joint injuries. Simple balance exercises (like standing on one leg or using a balance board) under supervision can be included in a physiotherapy regimen.
- *Activity pacing:* A unique concept in fibromyalgia/CFS management is pacing—distributing activity with appropriate rest to avoid overexertion crashes [19]. Patients are taught to "start low and go slow." For instance, if a patient can currently only manage 5 minutes of walking before pain worsens, they might do just 4 minutes twice a day and slowly increase by 1 minute every few days. If they have a day of heavier activity (like housework or a shopping trip), they are advised to follow it with a lighter day to recover. Keeping an activity log or using a pedometer/fitness tracker can help patients and clinicians set baselines and realistic incremental goals.

It is important to address patients' fear that exercise will worsen their pain. Many recall episodes where they tried to exercise, only to be bed-bound the next day. This is where patient education and physiotherapy guidance come in: distinguishing a normal transient increase in soreness from a pain flare and adjusting the plan accordingly. A well-versed physiotherapist or exercise therapist can be invaluable, especially early on, to craft a personalised exercise programme and supervise progress. In fibromyalgia, graded and individualised physical activity can be helpful. In ME/CFS, particularly where post-exertional malaise is present, activity should be paced carefully within the patient's energy limits and should not be increased irrespective of symptoms.

Cognitive Behavioural Therapy and Psychological Support

Given the interplay of the mind and body in chronic pain, addressing the psychological aspects is crucial. Cognitive behavioural therapy (CBT) is the most widely studied psychological intervention for fibromyalgia and chronic pain [20]. CBT aims to identify and modify negative thought patterns and behaviours that can exacerbate pain experience, for example, "catastrophising" (thinking the worst about pain) or avoidance of activity due to fear of pain. By restructuring thoughts (e.g. fostering more adaptive coping thoughts like "Even if I have pain, I can still engage in meaningful activities") and gradually increasing exposure to activity, CBT can reduce the emotional distress associated with pain and improve function.

Studies have shown CBT yields modest but meaningful improvements in fibromyalgia symptoms and coping ability [21]. It often leads to reduced pain behaviours, improved mood and a sense of empowerment in patients. For instance, a CBT programme might teach relaxation techniques, problem-solving skills for managing flare-ups, sleep hygiene education and goal-setting for activity [20]. Patients learn how stress and pain influence each other and develop strategies to interrupt this cycle (such as deep breathing or mindfulness when pain spikes instead of panicking). Some programmes incorporate *graded activity* within the CBT framework, helping patients gradually increase activities they have been avoiding.

It is worth noting that psychological interventions are not about "treating a psychiatric illness instead of fibromyalgia" but rather about treating the *whole person*. Chronic pain inherently has psychological impacts and components. Unfortunately, some patients are resistant to the suggestion of therapy, interpreting it as "the doctor thinks I'm crazy". This is where careful explanation is needed: emphasise that therapies like CBT are tools to help manage pain, not an insinuation that the pain is imaginary. Many patients, once they try it, find it does help them feel better and more in control.

Combining exercise with CBT or stress management often has a cumulative benefit. Indeed, some multidisciplinary programmes (often run in pain clinics or specialty rehab centres) provide a combination of supervised exercise, education sessions and group CBT over several weeks—the so-called "fibromyalgia day programmes" or pain rehabilitation programmes—which have shown improvements in overall function.

Pharmacotherapy

Medications can play a role in fibromyalgia and soft tissue pain management, chiefly to reduce symptom severity enough to engage in therapies like exercise. It is important to set the expectation that drugs typically yield partial relief (perhaps a 20–30% reduction in pain) in a subset of patients, rather than complete resolution [22]. Polypharmacy should be avoided; instead, choose medications targeting the patient's predominant symptoms (be it pain, poor sleep or mood issues). Below are the commonly used classes:

- *Tricyclic antidepressants (TCAs)* [23]: Low-dose amitriptyline (10–25 mg at night) is a long-standing first-line medication for fibromyalgia. Though an antidepressant at higher doses, at low doses, its effects are likely due to enhancement of descending pain inhibition via serotonin/norepinephrine and improving sleep architecture. Amitriptyline can help with pain and especially sleep quality. Cyclobenzaprine, a muscle relaxant structurally similar to TCAs, is often used as well (5–10 mg at night) with similar benefit in sleep and some pain relief. Side effects (anticholinergic effects like dry mouth, sedation and weight gain) can limit use, particularly in older patients or those with cardiac risk (amitriptyline can prolong QT interval). Nortriptyline (a TCA metabolite) sometimes is used as it may have slightly fewer side effects. Importantly, TCAs should usually be taken 2–3 hours before bedtime to capitalise on their sedative effect for sleep.
- *SNRIs (serotonin-norepinephrine reuptake inhibitors):* Duloxetine and milnacipran are two SNRIs that are FDA approved for fibromyalgia in some countries. They help modulate pain by increasing neurotransmitters that dampen pain

pathways. Duloxetine (commonly 30–60 mg daily) has demonstrated reductions in pain and improvements in function in fibromyalgia trials, particularly in patients with concurrent mood disorders [24]. It may also help with comorbid anxiety or depression. Milnacipran (up to 100 mg twice daily) similarly can reduce pain and improve fatigue and cognitive symptoms for some patients. These medications tend to be stimulating (can cause insomnia or jitteriness) in some people, so are usually given in the morning (milnacipran often split BID, duloxetine QAM). Common side effects are nausea, dry mouth, sweating and increased blood pressure or heart rate. Both duloxetine and milnacipran have shown a subset of patients (~30%) achieving at least 30% pain reduction, but many others have minimal response [24]. If one SNRI is not tolerated or effective, sometimes the other can be tried. Venlafaxine (another SNRI) is less studied in fibromyalgia but might help at higher doses that affect norepinephrine (≥150 mg).

- *α-2-δ Ligands (anticonvulsants)* [25]: Pregabalin and gabapentin, which calm neuronal hyperexcitability by modulating calcium channels, are frequently used. Pregabalin is FDA approved for fibromyalgia in the USA. It can reduce pain intensity and improve sleep in some patients. Typical dosing is 150–300 mg daily (split BID); some patients may require 450 mg/day. Gabapentin (off-label for fibromyalgia) in doses of 1200–2400 mg/day (split TID) has shown some efficacy too. These medications are particularly helpful if there is a prominent neuropathic pain component (e.g. burning, tingling) or marked sleep disturbance. They tend to cause sedation, dizziness, peripheral oedema and weight gain as side effects [25]. Starting low (e.g. 75 mg pregabalin at night or 100–300 mg gabapentin at night) and titrating slowly can improve tolerability. In practice, pregabalin/gabapentin help a subset of fibromyalgia patients quite a bit, while others get no benefit or cannot tolerate them.
- *Analgesics and NSAIDs* [24]: Simple analgesics like paracetamol can be used for temporary relief with minimal risk, though alone they often are not sufficient for fibromyalgia pain. Nonsteroidal anti-inflammatory drugs (NSAIDs), such as ibuprofen or naproxen, are commonly tried, especially if there's coexisting peripheral pain (like osteoarthritis or myofascial elements). However, in pure fibromyalgia, NSAIDs often provide little relief since there is no major inflammatory process—any benefit may be from general analgesic effect or placebo. They can still be used for symptomatic relief of headaches, menstrual pain, etc., but patients should be warned not to rely heavily on NSAIDs long term given gastrointestinal, renal and cardiovascular side effects. Topical NSAID creams or patches could be useful for focal myofascial pain spots (e.g. a painful trapezius area), with minimal systemic absorption.
- *Opioids:* Routine use of opioids in fibromyalgia is not recommended [26]. Studies and clinical experience have shown that classic opioids (like hydrocodone and oxycodone) often do not provide significant benefit in fibromyalgia and carry substantial risks (tolerance, dependence, opioid-induced hyperalgesia, side effects such as constipation and sedation).

- *Sleep aids* [27]: Sleep is a major target. If low-dose amitriptyline does not sufficiently help sleep, short-term hypnotics may occasionally be considered for severe insomnia, but they should not be routine fibromyalgia treatment and carry risks of tolerance, dependence, falls and next-day impairment. However, these do not treat pain and can lead to dependence or next-day drowsiness, so they are a second line for resistant insomnia. Melatonin supplementation might help regulate sleep in some cases and has antioxidant properties; it is benign to try. Gabapentin or pregabalin at night can also improve sleep depth in patients who tolerate it, thus serving dual purpose for pain and sleep.

Combination therapy is common—for example, a patient may be on a low-dose TCA at night and duloxetine in the morning. This can target different mechanisms (sleep vs daytime pain). However, be cautious with combining multiple serotonergic drugs (risk of serotonin syndrome, albeit rare at low doses—for example, combining TCA + SNRI + tramadol would stack serotonergic effects—such combinations should be monitored closely or avoided).

It is also prudent to periodically reevaluate the medication regimen. If a drug is not helping after an adequate trial (say 2–3 months at therapeutic dose), it should be tapered and stopped to reduce polypharmacy. Similarly, if the patient has improved and been stable, a trial of tapering medications can be considered to see if they are still needed. Pharmacotherapy in fibromyalgia is aimed at symptom control to facilitate engagement in non-pharmacologic therapies. It should rarely be the sole treatment.

Other Non-pharmacological Modalities

Physiotherapy and occupational therapy [2]: A skilled physiotherapist can provide tailored stretching and strengthening regimens, manual therapy (such as myofascial release or gentle massage to taut bands) and modalities like TENS (transcutaneous electrical nerve stimulation) or hydrotherapy. While passive modalities alone (ultrasound, heat packs, etc.) have limited lasting effect, they can be useful adjuncts to reduce pain enough for the patient to then exercise. Occupational therapists can help patients with energy conservation techniques, ergonomic advice (setting up home/work environment to reduce strain) and assistive devices if needed (like splints or braces for hypermobile joints during certain activities).

Trigger point injections and dry needling [28]: For patients with prominent myofascial trigger points, targeted therapy can help. Dry needling involves inserting a thin needle (acupuncture-like) into trigger points to elicit a twitch response and relieve the contraction knot. It can reduce local pain and referred pain temporarily. Adding a small amount of local anaesthetic (0.5% lidocaine, for instance) turns it into a trigger point injection. Some patients get relief for days to weeks from such interventions, which can be repeated periodically. However, addressing the underlying contributors (postural issues, stress, etc.) is needed for sustained improvement.

Acupuncture [29]: Traditional Chinese acupuncture has shown mixed but generally positive results in fibromyalgia trials. Some patients respond well in terms of pain reduction and relaxation. Given its low risk, a course of acupuncture can be considered for interested patients. It may function via endogenous opioid release or simply as a novel sensory input that modulates pain pathways.

Massage therapy [30]: Gentle massage can temporarily reduce muscle tension and anxiety, improving well-being. A regular schedule (e.g. monthly massage) might help some patients as part of their self-care, though lasting effects on pain are variable. Deep aggressive massages are usually not tolerated; a knowledgeable massage therapist experienced with fibromyalgia can be an asset.

Heat and hydrotherapy [31]: Superficial heat (hot showers, warm baths, heating pads) often soothes achy muscles and can be used daily, especially in morning to loosen stiffness. Warm water therapy combines buoyancy and heat—many fibromyalgia patients report significant short-term relief after a session. Saunas or steam rooms might similarly help, though hydration must be maintained.

Transcranial magnetic stimulation (TMS) and other neuromodulation [32]: These are more experimental in fibromyalgia. TMS, an FDA-approved treatment for depression, has been explored for fibromyalgia pain with some studies showing modest benefits on pain and mood. Similarly, transcranial direct current stimulation (tDCS) is being researched. These are not standard care yet but represent the frontier of trying to recalibrate neural networks in chronic pain.

Dietary approaches [33]: No specific diet cures fibromyalgia, but some patients explore anti-inflammatory diets (rich in fruits, vegetables and omega-3 fatty acids) or elimination diets if they suspect certain foods worsen symptoms (e.g. some find reducing caffeine or artificial sweeteners helps sleep or headaches). While evidence is scant, general healthy eating should be encouraged. Obesity exacerbates pain via increased load and proinflammatory adipokines, so weight management through diet and exercise can improve overall pain levels over time.

Supplements [34]: A variety of supplements have been tried (magnesium, malic acid, CoQ10, omega-3, vitamins, etc.) with inconsistent results. Vitamin D is worth supplementing if low. Otherwise, patients can be informed that most supplements lack strong evidence, but if one is safe and they wish to try (and it is not overly expensive), it could be a personal trial.

The management of fibromyalgia is highly individualised. A useful approach is to create a multidisciplinary plan possibly with input from a rheumatologist (for diagnosis and overall coordination), a physiotherapist, a psychologist or pain counsellor and the primary care provider for ongoing support. Some patients benefit from a pain clinic programme if available, which often combines many of the above strategies in a structured way.

Crucially, patient engagement in the treatment plan is what determines success. The patient should feel like an active participant rather than a passive recipient. This means collaborative goal setting (what activities do they want to get back to?), discussing preferences (some may be more willing to try therapy than meds, or vice versa, so adjust order accordingly) and continuous encouragement.

Role of Rheumatologists and Referral Thresholds

Referral thresholds for fibromyalgia and soft tissue pain can be considered at two levels: referral to rheumatology and referral from rheumatology to other specialists:

- *When should a patient be referred to rheumatology?* Generally, if a patient has chronic widespread pain (>3 months) that is unexplained, especially with any positive screening tests (like an ANA) or subtle signs that could indicate an autoimmune rheumatic disease, a referral ought to be considered.
  Primary care doctors often refer when inflammatory markers are elevated or if the patient has significant joint stiffness or swelling concerns. Another scenario is when the primary provider is uncertain or uncomfortable diagnosing fibromyalgia and wants a specialist confirmation. If a patient clearly meets fibromyalgia criteria and has no red flags, one might argue a confident primary care physician could manage them without referral, but often both patient and doctor feel more reassured after a rheumatology evaluation. Additionally, if initial fibromyalgia management by the GP fails or the patient has severe symptoms, a rheumatology referral for more advanced management advice is reasonable.
- *Rheumatology to other referrals:* Rheumatologists might involve other professionals once the diagnosis is made:
  - *Physiotherapy:* Almost all fibromyalgia patients should be referred to physiotherapy or instructed on exercise. Many rheumatology clinics have allied physios on team or can prescribe a course of PT to educate the patient on an exercise regimen.
  - *Pain management specialist:* If a patient's pain remains severe despite first-line treatments, or if they require interventions like trigger point injections, a pain specialist consultation can be useful. Pain clinics often take on fibromyalgia patients for multidisciplinary programmes. Also, if there is consideration of more exotic treatments (like infusion therapies or neurostimulation), pain specialists are the ones involved.
  - *Psychology/psychiatry:* Referral to a psychologist for CBT, or to a psychiatrist if mood disorders are prominent and not adequately managed, is common. For instance, a fibromyalgia patient with major depression might benefit from a psychiatrist adjusting medications or providing therapy beyond what the rheumatologist can do in limited visits.
  - *Sleep specialist:* If severe sleep apnoea or other primary sleep disorder is suspected (e.g. heavy snoring, witnessed apnoeas or restless legs not controlled), a sleep medicine referral for a sleep study and targeted treatment can dramatically help fatigue and pain in those cases.
  - *Sport and exercise medicine:* If alongside fibromyalgia there is a distinct musculoskeletal issue (like rotator cuff tear or knee osteoarthritis) that might benefit from intervention, a referral is appropriate. Fibromyalgia does not preclude coexisting focal musculoskeletal pathology, and new focal symptoms should be assessed on their own merits. However, caution: some

fibromyalgia patients get multiple surgical or invasive procedures in hopes of cure, which often do not help the overall pain (e.g. widespread pain rarely improves by an orthopaedic surgery on one area, and surgeries can sometimes even trigger worse fibromyalgia flares due to stress).

Other rheumatology referrals: If a patient with fibromyalgia also has signs of hypermobility or possible Ehlers-Danlos syndrome, referral to a clinical geneticist or a specialised hypermobility clinic might be done by the rheumatologist for confirmation and additional guidance.

In terms of continued rheumatology follow-up, practices vary. Some rheumatologists follow fibromyalgia patients long term, especially if they run a fibromyalgia clinic or if the patient has nowhere else to coordinate care. Others might see the patient for 1–3 visits to confirm diagnosis and initiate treatment and then discharge back to primary care with a management plan. The decision often depends on resource availability and patient needs. If the patient is improving and the GP is comfortable continuing the plan, follow-up can be with GP. If the patient has refractory symptoms or prefers specialist oversight, the rheumatologist might see them periodically. Additionally, if the patient has concomitant rheumatic diseases (e.g. a patient with lupus or rheumatoid arthritis *and* fibromyalgia, which is common), then rheumatology will continue managing the primary rheumatic disease, and fibromyalgia is addressed in parallel.

For hypermobility syndrome patients, a rheumatologist might coordinate with physiotherapists and sometimes geneticists (for EDS), and refer to pain specialists if needed for chronic pain. For myofascial pain syndrome, rheumatologists sometimes perform trigger point injections or refer to pain clinics for those procedures if needed.

In conclusion, rheumatologists play a pivotal role in the evaluation and initial management of generalised soft tissue pain syndromes like fibromyalgia. They determine if there is "any fire behind the smoke" of reported symptoms—that is, an autoimmune or inflammatory cause—and when it's fibromyalgia, they turn the focus to symptom management and rehabilitation. Determining appropriate referrals (to allied health or other specialists) ensures comprehensive care. Primary care remains extremely important for long-term follow-up, and good communication between rheumatologist and GP will benefit the patient greatly.

Key Learning Points

- Fibromyalgia is a common cause of chronic widespread musculoskeletal pain, defined by central sensitisation. It presents with diffuse pain, fatigue, unrefreshing sleep and cognitive, often accompanied by headaches, irritable bowel syndrome and mood disturbances.
- Myofascial pain syndrome is a localised soft tissue pain disorder characterised by trigger points in muscle—taut bands with focal tenderness and referred pain. It is distinguished from fibromyalgia by its regional distribution and the presence

of trigger points on exam, although fibromyalgia and myofascial pain often coexist.

- Joint hypermobility syndrome (and hypermobile EDS) can cause chronic pain due to joint laxity and microinjuries. There is significant overlap between hypermobility syndromes and fibromyalgia—many patients fulfil criteria for both, suggesting shared mechanisms like central sensitisation from chronic nociceptive input.
- Fibromyalgia commonly overlaps with other functional syndromes such as chronic fatigue syndrome (ME/CFS), IBS, tension headaches and temporomandibular disorder. These "central sensitivity syndromes" share symptoms and pathophysiology. An integrated approach addressing all symptoms is more effective than treating each in isolation.
- Patient education and reassurance are fundamental in fibromyalgia management. Validating the patient's pain, explaining the neurophysiological basis (e.g. pain amplification) and setting realistic expectations improve engagement and reduce anxiety.
- Exercise is the most evidence-backed treatment for fibromyalgia. Regular aerobic exercise (land or water-based) and gentle strength training improve pain, function and well-being. The key is gradual, paced introduction of activity to avoid flares, often under guidance of physiotherapy.
- Cognitive behavioural therapy (CBT) and related psychological interventions help patients develop coping strategies, reframe negative thoughts and address stress, which can lead to modest improvements in pain and significant gains in quality of life.
- Medications can be used to target key symptoms: low-dose tricyclics (amitriptyline) for sleep and pain, SNRIs (duloxetine, milnacipran) for pain and mood and gabapentinoids (pregabalin, gabapentin) for pain and sleep modulation. These drugs typically provide partial relief; a combination may be needed, but avoid polypharmacy and opioids if possible.
- Building a strong therapeutic alliance is crucial. Fibromyalgia patients often feel stigmatised. Empathy, consistent follow-up and open communication help rebuild trust. Acknowledge the reality of their illness and collaborate on a management plan tailored to their life context.
- Rheumatologists are key in diagnosing fibromyalgia and excluding other rheumatic diseases. Once fibromyalgia is diagnosed, a multidisciplinary management plan should be implemented, often in coordination with primary care. Rheumatology follow-up is individualised; many patients can be co-managed or primarily managed by their GP after the initial workup and advice.
- Timely referrals to physiotherapy, pain specialists, mental health professionals or other specialists (e.g. sport and exercise medicine if needed) should be made based on each patient's predominant issues. For example, refractory pain may benefit from pain clinic input (injections, pain programmes), and severe psychosocial distress may warrant psychology/psychiatry involvement.
- The overall goal of management is to improve function and quality of life rather than to eliminate pain entirely. Success is measured in the patient regaining

abilities and confidence—for example, returning to work or hobbies, sleeping better and self-managing flare-ups effectively—even if some pain persists at a tolerable level.

References

1. Bhargava J, Goldin J. Fibromyalgia [Internet]. StatPearls. 2026. Available from: http://www.ncbi.nlm.nih.gov/pubmed/26379048.
2. Antunes MD, Marques AP. The role of physiotherapy in fibromyalgia: current and future perspectives. Front Physiol [Internet]. 2022;13. Available from: https://www.frontiersin.org/articles/10.3389/fphys.2022.968292/full.
3. Vincent A, Benzo RP, Whipple MO, McAllister SJ, Erwin PJ, Saligan LN. Beyond pain in fibromyalgia: insights into the symptom of fatigue. Arthritis Res Ther [Internet]. 2013;15(6):221. Available from: http://www.ncbi.nlm.nih.gov/pubmed/24289848.
4. Dua A, Chang K-V. Myofascial pain syndrome [Internet]. StatPearls. 2026. Available from: http://www.ncbi.nlm.nih.gov/pubmed/25135034.
5. Syx D, De Wandele I, Rombaut L, Malfait F. Hypermobility, the Ehlers-Danlos syndromes and chronic pain. Clin Exp Rheumatol [Internet]. 2017;35 Suppl 1(5):116–22. Available from: http://www.ncbi.nlm.nih.gov/pubmed/28967365.
6. Carroll MB. Hypermobility spectrum disorders: a review. Rheumatol Immunol Res [Internet]. 2023;4(2):60–8. Available from: http://www.ncbi.nlm.nih.gov/pubmed/37637226.
7. Di Stefano G, Celletti C, Baron R, Castori M, Di Franco M, La Cesa S, et al. Central sensitization as the mechanism underlying pain in joint hypermobility syndrome/Ehlers-Danlos syndrome, hypermobility type. Eur J Pain [Internet]. 2016;20(8):1319–25. Available from: http://www.ncbi.nlm.nih.gov/pubmed/26919608.
8. Häuser W, Fitzcharles M-A, Henningsen P. Fibromyalgia syndrome-a bodily distress disorder/somatic symptom disorder? Pain Rep [Internet]. 2025;10(1):e1223. Available from: http://www.ncbi.nlm.nih.gov/pubmed/39816901.
9. Kumbhare D, Hassan S, Diep D, Duarte FCK, Hung J, Damodara S, et al. Potential role of blood biomarkers in patients with fibromyalgia: a systematic review with meta-analysis. Pain [Internet]. 2022;163(7):1232–53. Available from: http://www.ncbi.nlm.nih.gov/pubmed/34966131.
10. Malek S, Reinhold EJ, Pearce GS. The Beighton score as a measure of generalised joint hypermobility. Rheumatol Int [Internet]. 2021;41(10):1707–16. Available from: http://www.ncbi.nlm.nih.gov/pubmed/33738549.
11. D'Amuri A, Greco S, Pagani M, Presciuttini B, Ciaffi J, Ursini F. Common non-rheumatic medical conditions mimicking fibromyalgia: a simple framework for differential diagnosis. Diagnostics (Basel, Switzerland) [Internet]. 2024;14(16). Available from: http://www.ncbi.nlm.nih.gov/pubmed/39202246.
12. Scott L, Dolan E, Baker N, Melia Y. Exploring attitudes of healthcare professionals towards those with fibromyalgia: a Q-methodological approach. Br J Pain [Internet]. 2023;17(4):352–65. Available from: http://www.ncbi.nlm.nih.gov/pubmed/37538944.
13. Romano GF, Tomassi S, Russell A, Mondelli V, Pariante CM. Fibromyalgia and chronic fatigue: the underlying biology and related theoretical issues. Adv Psychosom Med [Internet]. 2015;34:61–77. Available from: http://www.ncbi.nlm.nih.gov/pubmed/25832514.
14. White KP, Speechley M, Harth M, Ostbye T. Co-existence of chronic fatigue syndrome with fibromyalgia syndrome in the general population. A controlled study. Scand J Rheumatol [Internet]. 2000;29(1):44–51. Available from: http://www.ncbi.nlm.nih.gov/pubmed/10722257.

15. Climent-Sanz C, Hamilton KR, Martínez-Navarro O, Briones-Vozmediano E, Gracia-Lasheras M, Fernández-Lago H, et al. Fibromyalgia pain management effectiveness from the patient perspective: a qualitative evidence synthesis. Disabil Rehabil [Internet]. 2024;46(20):4595–610. Available from: http://www.ncbi.nlm.nih.gov/pubmed/37965900.
16. Jones EA, Asaad F, Patel N, Jain E, Abd-Elsayed A. Management of fibromyalgia: an update. Biomedicines [Internet]. 2024;12(6). Available from: http://www.ncbi.nlm.nih.gov/pubmed/38927473.
17. Macfarlane GJ, Kronisch C, Dean LE, Atzeni F, Häuser W, Fluß E, et al. EULAR revised recommendations for the management of fibromyalgia. Ann Rheum Dis [Internet]. 2017;76(2):318–28. Available from: http://www.ncbi.nlm.nih.gov/pubmed/27377815.
18. Wang C, Schmid CH, Fielding RA, Harvey WF, Reid KF, Price LL, et al. Effect of tai chi versus aerobic exercise for fibromyalgia: comparative effectiveness randomized controlled trial. BMJ [Internet]. 2018;360:k851. Available from: http://www.ncbi.nlm.nih.gov/pubmed/29563100
19. Sanal-Hayes NEM, Mclaughlin M, Hayes LD, Mair JL, Ormerod J, Carless D, et al. A scoping review of "Pacing" for management of Myalgic Encephalomyelitis/Chronic Fatigue Syndrome (ME/CFS): lessons learned for the long COVID pandemic. J Transl Med [Internet]. 2023;21(1):720. Available from: http://www.ncbi.nlm.nih.gov/pubmed/37838675.
20. Bernardy K, Klose P, Busch AJ, Choy EHS, Häuser W. Cognitive behavioural therapies for fibromyalgia. Cochrane Database Syst Rev [Internet]. 2013;2013(9):CD009796. Available from: http://www.ncbi.nlm.nih.gov/pubmed/24018611.
21. Menga G, Ing S, Khan O, Dupre B, Dornelles AC, Alarakhia A, et al. Fibromyalgia: can online cognitive behavioral therapy help? Ochsner J [Internet]. 2014;14(3):343–9. Available from: http://www.ncbi.nlm.nih.gov/pubmed/25249800.
22. Giorgi V, Sarzi-Puttini P, Pellegrino G, Sirotti S, Atzeni F, Alciati A, et al. Pharmacological treatment of fibromyalgia syndrome: a practice-based review. Curr Pain Headache Rep [Internet]. 2024;28(12):1349–63. Available from: http://www.ncbi.nlm.nih.gov/pubmed/39042299.
23. Moore RA, Derry S, Aldington D, Cole P, Wiffen PJ. Amitriptyline for fibromyalgia in adults. Cochrane Database Syst Rev [Internet]. 2019;5(7):CD011824. Available from: http://www.ncbi.nlm.nih.gov/pubmed/35658166.
24. Häuser W, Walitt B, Fitzcharles M-A, Sommer C. Review of pharmacological therapies in fibromyalgia syndrome. Arthritis Res Ther [Internet]. 2014;16(1):201. Available from: https://arthritis-research.biomedcentral.com/articles/10.1186/ar4441.
25. Derry S, Cording M, Wiffen PJ, Law S, Phillips T, Moore RA. Pregabalin for pain in fibromyalgia in adults. Cochrane Database Syst Rev [Internet]. 2016;9(9):CD011790. Available from: http://www.ncbi.nlm.nih.gov/pubmed/27684492.
26. Hurtado I, Robles C, Peiró S, García-Sempere A, Llopis F, Sánchez F, et al. Long versus short-term opioid therapy for fibromyalgia syndrome and risk of depression, sleep disorders and suicidal ideation: a population-based, propensity-weighted cohort study. RMD Open [Internet]. 2024;10(3). Available from: http://www.ncbi.nlm.nih.gov/pubmed/39313306.
27. Pathak A, Kelleher EM, Brennan I, Amarnani R, Wall A, Murphy R, et al. Treatments for enhancing sleep quality in fibromyalgia: a systematic review and meta-analysis. Rheumatology (Oxford) [Internet]. 2025;64(8):4495–516. Available from: http://www.ncbi.nlm.nih.gov/pubmed/40084994
28. Hammi C, Schroeder JD, Yeung B. Trigger point injection [Internet]. StatPearls. 2026. Available from: http://www.ncbi.nlm.nih.gov/pubmed/17321283.
29. Berger AA, Liu Y, Nguyen J, Spraggins R, Reed DS, Lee C, et al. Efficacy of acupuncture in the treatment of fibromyalgia. Orthop Rev (Pavia) [Internet]. 2021;13(2):25085. Available from: http://www.ncbi.nlm.nih.gov/pubmed/34745475.
30. Kalichman L. Massage therapy for fibromyalgia symptoms. Rheumatol Int [Internet]. 2010;30(9):1151–7. Available from: http://www.ncbi.nlm.nih.gov/pubmed/20306046.
31. Chadwick AL, Shi C, McMillan M, Miller J, Hu J, Geiger PC. The impact of a heat therapy intervention on pain and fibromyalgia symptoms in patients with fibromyalgia: a pilot

study. Front Pain Res (Lausanne, Switzerland) [Internet]. 2025;6:1526491. Available from: http://www.ncbi.nlm.nih.gov/pubmed/40182803
32. Sun P, Fang L, Zhang J, Liu Y, Wang G, Qi R. Repetitive transcranial magnetic stimulation for patients with fibromyalgia: a systematic review with meta-analysis. Pain Med [Internet]. 2022;23(3):499–514. Available from: http://www.ncbi.nlm.nih.gov/pubmed/34542624.
33. Kadayifci FZ, Bradley MJ, Onat AM, Shi HN, Zheng S. Review of nutritional approaches to fibromyalgia. Nutr Rev [Internet]. 2022;80(12):2260–74. Available from: http://www.ncbi.nlm.nih.gov/pubmed/35674686.
34. Haddad HW, Mallepalli NR, Scheinuk JE, Bhargava P, Cornett EM, Urits I, et al. The role of nutrient supplementation in the management of chronic pain in fibromyalgia: a narrative review. Pain Ther [Internet]. 2021;10(2):827–48. Available from: http://www.ncbi.nlm.nih.gov/pubmed/33909266.

Management Strategies and Rehabilitation Principles

12

Abstract

Effective management of soft tissue rheumatic conditions requires an integrative, patient-centred approach. This chapter brings together core principles of treating musculoskeletal soft tissue pain, building on concepts from previous chapters. We explore general strategies including patient education, exercise prescription, physiotherapy modalities and the use of interventions like injection therapy. The importance of tailored exercise (aerobic, strengthening and flexibility training) and progressive rehabilitation is emphasised as a means to restore function and prevent recurrence. We discuss injection therapies (e.g. corticosteroid, hyaluronic acid)—their indications, benefits and risks—and outline when referral to orthopaedic surgery or pain specialists is warranted for advanced care. Strategies for preventing recurrent injuries and flares are highlighted, along with the construction of a patient-centred management plan that aligns with individual goals and addresses psychosocial factors. Finally, we address "red flags" that may signal a more serious underlying issue and common pitfalls in treatment to avoid. The overarching aim is to provide a framework for comprehensive rehabilitation of patients with soft tissue and musculoskeletal pain, ensuring evidence-based practice and optimal outcomes.

Integrative Summary of Soft Tissue Management Strategies

Soft tissue rheumatism encompasses a variety of conditions—tendinopathies (tendonitis, tendinosis), bursitis, enthesopathies, myofascial pain, ligament sprains, etc. Despite differences in anatomic location or tissue involved, the overarching management principles share common threads. Treatment must often address pain relief, inflammation control (if present), mechanical factors and functional restoration. Moreover, these conditions exist within the biopsychosocial context of the patient,

© The Author(s), under exclusive license to Springer Nature Switzerland AG 2026
R. Amarnani, *Soft Tissue and Musculoskeletal Medicine in Rheumatology*,
https://doi.org/10.1007/978-3-032-29441-8_12

meaning that psychological and social considerations (like fear of movement or job demands) influence outcomes and must be integrated into management.

An integrative management strategy means combining multiple modalities and tailoring them to the patient's specific condition, needs and preferences. Typically, management can be divided into:

- *Conservative measures:* relative rest or activity modification, ice/heat, compression and bracing
- *Rehabilitative measures:* physiotherapy, exercise and manual therapy
- *Pharmacological measures:* analgesics, NSAIDs or other medications to alleviate pain/inflammation
- *Interventional measures:* injections and minimally invasive procedures if indicated
- *Educational and preventive measures:* patient education on their condition, ergonomics, posture and strategies to prevent recurrence
- *Surgical measures:* reserved for cases that do not respond to the above or where structural pathology requires correction

A key concept is the stepwise approach. Often initial treatment is conservative and symptomatic; if that fails, one escalates to more invasive interventions. For example, in lateral epicondylitis (tennis elbow), one might start with activity modification and exercises; if pain persists, reassess the diagnosis and loading programme, consider options such as bracing, physiotherapy progression, shockwave therapy or selected injection options; corticosteroid may provide short-term relief but should be used cautiously.

Multidisciplinary collaboration is a hallmark of effective soft tissue pain management. The sports medicine physician or rheumatologist might coordinate care with physiotherapists, occupational therapists, orthopaedic surgeons, pain specialists and others as needed. This ensures that all aspects, from physical reconditioning to psychosocial support, are addressed.

Important general principles include the following:

- *Early mobilisation (with protection):* Prolonged immobilisation of soft tissue injuries can lead to stiffness, muscle atrophy and delayed healing [1]. Except in acute tears or fractures that necessitate immobilisation, most soft tissue injuries benefit from early gentle motion [2]. The adage "rest to recover, but don't rust" applies. For instance, in subacute low back pain, bed rest beyond a day or two is detrimental; staying active within pain limits speeds recovery.
- *Inflammation control:* In conditions with an acute inflammatory component (like bursitis or tendonitis), addressing inflammation helps pain and facilitates rehabilitation. This may involve NSAIDs, ice and sometimes steroid injection (for focal intense inflammation). However, many chronic soft tissue pains (like tendinosis) are more degenerative than inflammatory, so anti-inflammatory measures alone will not solve the problem and the focus should shift to tissue remodelling strategies (e.g. eccentric exercise for tendinopathy) [3].

- *Mechanical offloading vs strengthening:* There is often a dual need to offload the injured tissue to allow recovery *and* to strengthen supporting structures to prevent recurrence. For example, consider Achilles tendinopathy. Initially, reducing high-impact activities (like running and jumping) and using heel lifts or supportive footwear offloads the tendon to let pain settle; concurrently or soon after, initiating a programme of eccentric calf strengthening is crucial to stimulate tendon repair and build resilience. Thus, management oscillates between protecting the tissue and gradually loading it [3].
- *Addressing contributing factors:* Many soft tissue conditions are precipitated or perpetuated by modifiable factors: poor ergonomics, muscle imbalances, improper sports techniques, obesity or footwear issues. A truly integrative approach identifies these and intervenes. For example, chronic neck-shoulder myofascial pain might be fuelled by an ergonomically poor workstation; adjusting chair height, monitoring position and encouraging microbreaks can relieve strain [4]. Plantar fasciitis may be aggravated by tight calf muscles and improper shoes; thus calf stretching and shoe orthotics are part of management.
- *Patient-centered goal setting:* A recreational runner with iliotibial band syndrome will have a different goal (return to running) compared to a sedentary office worker with the same condition (simply being pain-free during daily activities). Aligning the rehabilitation plan with what the patient values ensures motivation and relevance. Goals should be specific, measurable, achievable, relevant and time-bound (SMART).
- *Regular reassessment:* Soft tissue conditions typically evolve over time. What is appropriate in the acute phase (e.g. more rest, pain control) differs from what is needed in subacute (gradual loading) and chronic phases (advanced strengthening, return to sport training). Regular follow-up allows the clinician to adjust the programme. If progress is stalled, it triggers reevaluation of diagnosis (Did we miss a tear? Is there a biomechanical issue unaddressed?), adherence (Is the patient doing the exercises?) or psychosocial barriers (fear of pain, low mood interfering with engagement).
- *Education and self-management:* Patients should be educated about their condition's natural history and taught self-management techniques. For example, for recurrent tension-type neck pain, teach them a set of home stretching and strengthening exercises, use of a heat pack for flare-ups and stress management techniques. The patient thus gains tools to manage minor recurrences independently, seeking professional help only if needed. This empowerment is crucial in conditions prone to flare-ups.

Ultimately, integrating these strategies leads to a comprehensive plan that not only treats the current issue but also reduces risk of future injury. Now, we will delve into specific components of this integrated approach: physiotherapy principles, exercise prescription, injection therapies, indications for specialist referral, prevention strategies, patient-centred planning and red flags/pitfalls.

Core Principles of Physiotherapy and Rehabilitation

Physiotherapy is central to restoring function in musculoskeletal conditions. The core principles revolve around relieving pain, restoring mobility, strengthening and improving functional performance. Key principles include the following:

1. *Pain modulation:* Early in rehabilitation, controlling pain is necessary to allow participation in therapy. Physiotherapists employ various modalities for this:
   - *Thermal modalities:* Superficial heat (hot packs, warm water baths) helps reduce muscle spasm and improve blood flow, easing pain and stiffness. Cold therapy (ice packs) is typically used in acute injury or after exercise if inflammation is present, to reduce swelling and numb pain.
   - *Electrotherapy* [5]: TENS (transcutaneous electrical nerve stimulation) can provide short-term pain relief by stimulating nerve fibres and interfering with pain signalling. It is non-invasive and patients can even use home TENS units. Other modalities like ultrasound therapy or interferential current have been used, though evidence for ultrasound's long-term benefit in soft tissue injuries is limited [6]. They might provide temporary relief or placebo effect but should not be the sole focus.
   - *Manual therapy* [7]: Hands-on techniques such as massage, trigger point release or joint mobilisations can modulate pain and improve mobility. For example, gentle mobilisation of a frozen shoulder can increase range and reduce pain guarding. Myofascial release techniques can alleviate taut muscle bands contributing to pain.
   - *Dry needling/acupuncture* [8]: Some physiotherapists are trained in dry needling (inserting needles into trigger points) which can inactivate those points and reduce pain, as described earlier. Acupuncture (often with electric stimulation, "electroacupuncture") may also be applied by physiotherapists for pain relief in chronic low back pain, knee arthritis, etc., with some evidence of efficacy.
   - *Neuromuscular techniques* [9]: For pain exacerbated by muscle tension, techniques like strain-counterstrain or muscle energy techniques can help reset muscle tone. For instance, muscle energy technique in the neck (gentle isometric contractions followed by stretching) can relieve tension and pain.

These pain-focused interventions are usually the early-phase strategies—to calm the situation and allow progression to active therapy. It is important to transition to active therapy as soon as feasible, as passive modalities alone do not produce lasting improvements.

2. *Restoration of mobility and flexibility* [10]: Many soft tissue conditions lead to reduced range of motion (ROM) in joints or tightness in muscles:
   - *Stretching exercises:* Aimed at the muscles/tendons that are shortened or in spasm. Stretches can be static (holding a position for ~30 seconds) or dynamic

(controlled movement through range). In a post-immobilisation scenario (like after a cast removal), stretching helps regain lost ROM.

- *Joint mobilisation/manipulation*: Therapists may perform graded mobilisations on stiff joints. For instance, after shoulder injury, glenohumeral joint mobilisations can gradually improve abduction and rotation range. In the spine, mobilisation can reduce pain and improve mobility for facet joint dysfunction. Evidence supports that joint mobilisation can alleviate pain and improve ROM in conditions like adhesive capsulitis [11] or neck pain (with appropriate patient selection and avoiding manipulations in high-risk situations).
- *Postural correction:* Poor posture often contributes to muscle tightness and imbalance [12] (e.g. forward head posture causing neck and upper back strain). Physiotherapists work on posture through stretching tight anterior muscles (chest/neck flexors) and strengthening weak scapular muscles, as well as patient awareness (mirror feedback, ergonomic adjustments). Over time, improved posture reduces abnormal stress on soft tissues.
- *Soft tissue mobilisation:* Aside from stretching, therapists use techniques like transverse friction massage on tendons (like the common extensor tendon in tennis elbow) to mobilise scar tissue and possibly induce circulation for healing. In conditions like IT band syndrome, foam rolling or massage may reduce myofascial tightness in the lateral thigh.
- *Neural mobilisation:* Sometimes pain is exacerbated by neural tension (e.g. sciatica where hamstrings tighten and the sciatic nerve is less mobile). Nerve "glide" exercises gently mobilise nerves within their sheaths to reduce adhesions and sensitivity [13].

3. *Strengthening and muscle balance:* As pain subsides and mobility is regained, focus shifts to strengthening key muscle groups:
   - *Isometric to isotonic progression* [14]: Initially, if movement is painful or contraindicated, isometric exercises (muscle contraction without joint movement) can maintain some muscle activation (e.g. quadriceps sets after knee injury). As tolerated, isotonic exercises (through ROM, with or without resistance) are introduced. For example, for rotator cuff tendinopathy, once acute pain is controlled, begin with isometric external rotation exercises, and then progress to TheraBand or dumbbell-resisted exercises through range.
   - *Eccentric strengthening* [15]: For chronic tendinopathies, eccentric loading (lengthening contraction) has proven effective in stimulating tendon remodelling. Classic examples include eccentric calf drops for mid-portion Achilles tendinopathy and eccentric wrist extensor training for lateral epicondylitis. Eccentric exercise often initially causes some discomfort, but patients are instructed that mild pain is acceptable and to focus on slow, controlled motions. Over several weeks, eccentric training can reduce pain and improve tendon function, presumably by promoting collagen alignment and tensile strength.
   - *Core strength and stability* [16]: Many soft tissue pains, especially back pain, have a component of core weakness or poor lumbopelvic stability. Core exercises (targeting abdominal, paraspinal, gluteal and pelvic floor muscles) are

included to create a solid base for other movements. This can range from basic abdominal bracing exercises to advanced Pilates routines depending on the patient's level. Improved core strength reduces load on the spine and can prevent recurrence of back or pelvic injuries.

- *Scapular and joint stabilisers* [17]: For upper extremity issues, strengthening the scapular stabilisers (trapezius, serratus anterior, rhomboids) is crucial to proper shoulder mechanics, for example. In knee problems, strengthening the hip abductors and external rotators can offload the knee by improving alignment (especially in patellofemoral syndrome or IT band syndrome). Thus, rehabilitation often extends beyond the painful area to the kinetic chain—treating not just the "point of pain" but also proximal or distal muscle groups that influence biomechanics.
- *Proprioception and balance* [18]: Injury (like ankle sprains or ACL tears) can impair proprioception (the sense of joint position). Retraining balance and proprioception is key to preventing reinjury. For example, after an ankle sprain, doing single-leg stance exercises on an unstable surface (like a BOSU ball or balance board) helps retrain the peroneal muscles and balance reflexes, reducing risk of future sprains. Similarly, knee rehabilitation often includes balance and agility drills once basic strength is back, to simulate real-life challenges (cutting motions, uneven ground).
- *Functional strengthening:* Therapy should progress to mimic functional tasks. For an athlete, this might mean plyometric training (jumping, sprinting) when appropriate; for a manual labourer, it could mean simulated lifting tasks with proper body mechanics. This bridges the gap between isolated strengthening and actual real-world demands.

4. *Endurance and cardiovascular fitness:* Chronic pain patients often become deconditioned. Integrating aerobic exercise as part of rehabilitation is important not only for general health but also because improved aerobic fitness can reduce pain perception (via endorphin release and better oxygenation of tissues) [19]. Therapists may include cardiovascular components (stationary bike, treadmill walking, elliptical) at moderate intensity as tolerated. In subacute phases of an injury, non-impact cardio (like biking or swimming) can maintain fitness without stressing the injured part. For example, a runner with shin splints might do pool running or cycling to maintain cardio fitness while the tibial stress resolves. Once cleared, transferring that regained fitness to gradual running is easier than starting from scratch.
5. *Education and self-management:* Physiotherapists play a crucial educational role. They teach patients about the nature of their injury, healing timelines, pain vs harm (e.g. distinguishing the soreness of muscle use from damaging pain) and the importance of adherence to home exercise programmes. They also advise on ergonomics (how to lift correctly, how to set up a workstation, sleeping postures) and pacing of activities. A good physiotherapist ensures the patient leaves each session knowing exercises to practice at home—because what happens between sessions often matters more than the few hours a week in clinic. The ultimate

goal is to equip patients with the knowledge and exercises to manage their condition long-term.

6. *Gradual return to activity:* Rehabilitation is not complete until the patient has safely returned to their important daily activities, work or sports. Therapists often design a graded return-to-work plan or sports-specific drills. For example, for a soccer player with a hamstring strain, final rehabilitation stages involve sport-specific agility and sprint drills to ensure the hamstring can handle those demands. For a worker with low back pain, it might involve simulated lifting tasks and core endurance tests (like how long they can maintain a certain posture) to ensure readiness for job tasks.

In summary, physiotherapy takes a patient from acute injury through recovery to prevention of future injury by addressing pain, flexibility, strength and functional skills. It is tailored to the individual—a young athlete's programme will look very different from an older sedentary person's, even if both had, say, a rotator cuff tendinopathy. The principles, however, remain the same: relieve pain enough to engage the patient, and then progressively load tissues to stimulate healing and fortify the body, all while educating the patient on how to maintain improvements.

Exercise Prescription: Types, Dosing and Progression

Therapeutic exercise is a pillar of musculoskeletal rehabilitation. Crafting an exercise prescription involves selecting the right type of exercise, dosing it appropriately (frequency, intensity, duration) and progressing it over time as the patient improves. The exercise plan must be individualised, taking into account the patient's baseline fitness, specific condition and goals.

Types of Exercise [20]

- *Aerobic (endurance) exercise:* As discussed earlier, aerobic exercise improves cardiovascular fitness and has systemic benefits including reduced pain sensitivity and better mood. Aerobic exercise can also aid weight management, which is particularly important if excess weight is contributing to joint or tendon overload (e.g. knee osteoarthritis or plantar fasciitis). It is common to encourage at least 150 minutes of moderate-intensity aerobic exercise per week (per general health guidelines), but for someone in rehabilitation, this might be built up to gradually. For instance, start at 10 minutes of brisk walking three times a week and increase by 5 minutes each week as tolerated, up to target of 30 minutes five times a week.
- *Resistance (strength) training:* This includes weight training, resistance band exercises, bodyweight exercises, etc. It can be isotonic (movement through ROM) or isometric. For rehabilitation, the focus is usually on higher repetitions with lower weight initially (to build endurance and coordination) before heavier strength work if appropriate.
- *Flexibility (stretching) exercises:* These should ideally be done daily or almost daily. Stretching is often incorporated into warm-ups and cool-downs around

other exercises. There are static stretches (hold ~30 seconds, repeat a few times), dynamic stretches (moving stretches, often in warm-up) and PNF (proprioceptive neuromuscular facilitation) stretching which involves contraction-relaxation cycles that can enhance flexibility. It is important to ensure proper technique (slow, no bouncing in static stretching) and to avoid overstretching which can cause muscle fibre damage. Gains in flexibility help prevent injuries (e.g. tight calf muscles predispose to Achilles and plantar fascia problems, so regular calf stretches are preventive).

- *Neuromotor (balance/agility) training:* Especially relevant for older adults (to prevent falls) and athletes (to improve performance and prevent reinjury). Balance training might involve one-legged stands, using balance boards, agility ladder drills or sport-specific footwork. For an older patient with peripheral neuropathy causing unsteadiness, simple balance exercises can reduce fall risk. For an athlete, agility drills ensure they are ready to return to dynamic sports.
- *Functional and plyometric exercises:* Functional exercises mimic real-world tasks (like step-ups mimic stairs, sit-to-stand mimics getting out of a chair). These are excellent for bridging rehabilitation to daily life. Plyometrics (jumping, hopping, quick direction changes) are more advanced and usually reserved for athletic rehabilitation or later stages (e.g. rehabbing a basketball player's ankle sprain, eventually incorporating jumping drills to prepare for game situations).
- *Range-of-motion exercises:* These are sometimes listed separately—simply moving a joint through its available range. Early post-injury or surgery, active or passive ROM exercises prevent contractures and maintain joint mobility. For example, after shoulder surgery, pendulum exercises (gentle swinging of the arm) are given immediately to keep the joint from stiffening. As healing progresses, active ROM and eventually resisted ROM take over.

Dosing (Frequency, Intensity, Time) In exercise prescription, the FITT principle is commonly used [21]:

- *Frequency:* How often (days per week or times per day). For example, stretching might be daily, strengthening every other day for a muscle group, balance exercises three times/week, etc. Early rehabilitation might involve short sessions multiple times a day (like post-knee surgery doing ankle pumps and quad sets hourly to prevent clots and maintain activation). Later, a structured programme might be 3–4 days/week of combined exercises.
- *Intensity:* For aerobic exercise, intensity can be measured via heart rate (target heart rate zones), perceived exertion (Borg scale) or METs. In rehabilitation, an easy guide is that the exercise should be moderate (like brisk walk where talking is possible but you are slightly winded) unless training for higher athletic performance. For strengthening, intensity is often set by selecting a weight that allows the desired reps with some effort but not to complete failure initially. As a rule of thumb, many rehabilitation protocols use ~50–70% of one-rep max for 10–15

reps early on, possibly increasing intensity as tolerated. Or use body weight and increase reps until able to easily do >20, and then add resistance.

- *Time (duration):* For aerobic, how many minutes per session. For strength, it is more about sets and reps rather than continuous time. In chronic pain patients who are very deconditioned, even 5–10 minutes of exercise can be a starting goal, gradually building up by a few minutes each session. Duration should increase before intensity in fragile patients (first get them to tolerate sustained activity and then up the effort).
- *Type:* Covered above but ensure variety and address all relevant fitness domains.

Progression

- The progression should be gradual and guided by patient response. A general guideline is the "10% rule"—increase exercise volume by no more than ~10% per week to avoid overuse injuries. For instance, if a patient is walking 20 minutes per session, increase to 22 minutes, not 30, in the next week (which would be a 50% jump) [22].
- *Monitoring pain and fatigue:* Particularly in chronic pain or post-injury, if an increase in exercise leads to significant pain increase that does not settle in 24 hours, it might have been too much. Minor transient soreness (DOMS—delayed onset muscle soreness) is normal when progressing exercises, but sharp pain or joint swelling indicates overdoing. Patients should be taught to differentiate "muscle soreness" from "injury pain".
- *Phase-based progression:* Early phase (acute/subacute) focuses on mobility and gentle strengthening, mid-phase build strength and endurance, and late-phase works on advanced strength, power and return-to-activity drills. Criteria-based progression is best—the patient should meet certain milestones before advancing. For example, before a runner with stress fracture returns to running, they should be pain-free walking long distances, have full strength and no tenderness on exam.
- *Individual variation:* Some patients progress faster and others slower. A cookie-cutter approach can lead to frustration or reinjury. It is better to set *minimum* criteria (like "when you can do 3 sets of 15 heel raises without pain, we move to single-leg heel raises"). Achieving that might take one patient 2 weeks and another 4 weeks, and that is acceptable.
- *Periodisation for athletes:* Athletes may need a more formal progression plan with phases of training intensity and rest (like building base endurance, then adding strength, then power and then sport-specific drills). Even non-athletes benefit from variation—continually doing the exact same exercise routine may lead to plateau or boredom, so every few weeks some parameters are changed (increase weights, change exercises, incorporate intervals in cardio, etc.).
- *Supervision and feedback:* Early on, supervision by a physiotherapist or exercise physiologist is valuable to ensure proper form and progression. They can adjust exercises on the fly if too easy or too hard. As patients learn, they can do more on their own. Periodic check-ins ensure continued progression and troubleshoot any difficulties.

Special Considerations in Dosing and Progression [23]

- *Chronic pain/fibromyalgia:* For these patients, the motto is "low and slow". Even trivial-seeming exercise can trigger flares, so start well below what they think they can do, and increase in baby steps. Emphasise consistency (daily gentle movement) over intensity. Use time-based goals rather than intensity—for example, walk 10 minutes even if it is slow, rather than aim for a mile. Progress by minute increments.
- *Post-surgery or injury with healing tissues:* Must follow biological healing timelines. For example, after a rotator cuff repair, there is a protocol—often no active motion for some weeks (to protect the surgical repair), just passive movement and then active assisted, then active and then resistive exercises only after ~8–12 weeks when tendon healing is secure. Progression is slower because premature stress could retear tissue. Similarly, weight-bearing status after fractures or surgeries is often staged (nonweight-bearing to partial to full over weeks to months).
- *Children and adolescents:* Their tissues and growth plates need care—avoid excessive load that could damage growth plates (no max weight lifting until they have adequate musculoskeletal maturity). Emphasise technique and moderate reps vs heavy lifting. Progression can often be a bit faster in terms of healing, as younger tissues usually heal quicker but do not progress weight too rapidly to avoid overuse injuries.
- *Older adults:* Focus on higher reps and lower resistance initially to account for lower muscle mass and potential balance issues. Progression might be slower due to recovery times. But do not shy away from strength training in elders—evidence shows older adults can significantly improve muscle strength and bone density with progressive resistance training, which is crucial for maintaining independence.

In practice, documenting the exercise prescription and progression helps—for example, have the patient keep a log of what they did and their symptom response. This makes it easier to adjust next steps. It also motivates patients seeing improvements (like being able to do more this week than last)

Finally, always integrate rest/recovery into the programme. Muscles need recovery time after intense workouts—typically at least 48 hours before reworking the same muscle group heavily [24]. In rehabilitation, one might alternate days (upper body focus 1 day, lower body the next or active exercise 1 day and relative rest or gentle stretching the next). Adequate sleep and nutrition also play a role in how well patients progress with exercise; it is worth reminding them that good protein intake and hydration support tissue healing, and sleep is when a lot of recovery happens.

In summary, exercise prescription in MSK medicine is a thoughtful process that should adapt to the patient's condition, ensure safe but challenging progression and eventually lead the patient back to their desired activities stronger and more resilient than before.

Injection Therapy: Corticosteroids, Ultrasound Guidance and Indications

Injection therapies are a valuable tool in musculoskeletal medicine for both diagnosis and treatment. The most common injections are corticosteroid injections into joints or soft tissues, often combined with a local anaesthetic. Other injection modalities include prolotherapy, platelet-rich plasma (PRP), hyaluronic acid (for joints) and trigger point injections with anaesthetic. This section will focus primarily on corticosteroid injections, as they are widely used by rheumatologists and generalists for soft tissue conditions.

Mechanism of Corticosteroid Injections [25] Corticosteroids (such as methylprednisolone, triamcinolone or betamethasone) are potent anti-inflammatory agents. Injected locally, they reduce inflammation in the targeted tissue—whether that is a joint synovium, a swollen bursa or an inflamed tendon sheath. By curbing inflammation, they can break the cycle of pain and swelling, allowing the tissue to recover and the patient to engage in rehabilitation [25]. The addition of a local anaesthetic (like lidocaine) provides immediate pain relief and also serves a diagnostic purpose: if pain is substantially improved after local anaesthetic, this supports the targeted structure as a likely pain generator (e.g. a subacromial bursitis injection relieving shoulder pain suggests the bursa/impingement was the pain generator).

Common Indications for Steroid Injections [26]

- *Bursitis:* For example, subacromial bursitis (shoulder impingement syndrome), trochanteric bursitis (lateral hip pain) and olecranon bursitis (elbow). In bursitis, a well-placed steroid injection can dramatically reduce pain and swelling. For trochanteric bursitis, one injection often leads to significant relief and many patients may not need a repeat.
- *Tendon sheath inflammation (tenosynovitis):* For example, De Quervain's tenosynovitis (stenosing tenosynovitis of the first dorsal compartment at the wrist). Corticosteroid injection into the first dorsal compartment is highly effective and is often used when symptoms are moderate, persistent or not responding to splinting and activity modification, boasting a very high response rate (~83% in studies) [27] compared to splinting or NSAIDs. Trigger finger (flexor tendon pulley stenosis) is another example—a steroid injection near the pulley can often resolve the trigger without surgery.
- *Enthesopathy/plantar fasciopathy:* Corticosteroid injection can provide short-term relief in selected cases, but should be used cautiously because of risks such as plantar fascia rupture and fat pad atrophy.
- *Joint arthritis (intraarticular):* Though more a joint issue, many soft tissue pain patients also have OA or inflammatory arthritis. Intraarticular steroid injections in knee OA, for example, can reduce pain and improve function for 4–6 weeks on average [28]. Inflammatory arthritis flares (like a gouty arthritis or rheumatoid knee flare) are classic indications for joint injection to quickly reduce inflammation.

- *Nerve compressions:* Some peripheral entrapment neuropathies respond to injections, for example, carpal tunnel syndrome—a steroid injection into the carpal tunnel can shrink tenosynovium swelling and give temporary (or sometimes lasting) relief, delaying or avoiding surgery. Radiculopathy (like cervical or lumbar radicular pain from a herniated disc) can be managed with epidural steroid injections (often by pain specialists) to reduce nerve root inflammation.
- *Myofascial trigger points:* Trigger point injections (with or without steroid—usually just lidocaine but some add a tiny dose of steroid) can be done for persistent, extremely painful trigger points not releasing with other methods. However, steroid is not typically needed for pure trigger points—the needling and anaesthetic often can be enough [29].

Ultrasound Guidance The use of ultrasound (US) to guide injections has grown significantly. Ultrasound allows real-time visualisation of soft tissue structures, the needle and spread of injectate [30]. Benefits of US-guided injections are the following:

- *Accuracy:* Especially in small joints or when the target is near neurovascular structures, US ensures accurate placement.
- *Efficacy:* Some studies show improved outcomes when the injection is accurately placed [31, 32].
- *Safety:* Avoiding needle injury to nerves, vessels or tendon tissue is critical. US can identify, say, the median nerve in the carpal tunnel or large blood vessels in the path of a needle. For peritendinous steroid injections, ultrasound guidance helps inject around the tendon rather than into it, since intratendinous steroid can predispose to rupture.
- *Diagnostic info:* While scanning to guide, one might identify pathology (e.g. calcific deposits in a tendon, fluid in a bursa, partial tendon tear). This can refine diagnosis concurrently. Also, seeing the spread of the injectate confirms adequate coverage of the intended area.
- *Patient satisfaction:* Many patients appreciate the perceived precision, and often it is less painful since you can avoid multiple redirections by seeing exactly where to go [32].

Effectiveness and Limitations Steroid injections often provide short- to medium-term relief. This underscores that injections should usually be adjuncts, not standalone cures (except in some cases like De Quervain's where one injection often suffices). They create a window of pain relief during which the patient should do their rehabilitation exercises more effectively. In chronic conditions, repeated injections may be needed, but most guidelines limit this to protect tissues (commonly an empirical limit is no more than 3–4 injections per year in a given site, though evidence behind the exact number is sparse) [26].

Procedure and Aftercare Typically, injections are done with sterile technique. The area is identified (either by landmarks or US). The skin is cleaned with antiseptic; sometimes a topical anaesthetic or freeze spray is applied. A fine needle is used whenever possible. For example, injecting a finger tendon sheath might be done with a 25-gauge needle. The steroid dose depends on the area: large joints or bursae might get 40 mg of depot steroid (like triamcinolone acetonide); smaller areas like a carpal tunnel might get 10–20 mg. It is mixed with an appropriate amount of lidocaine/bupivacaine. When injecting, aspiration is done first to ensure not in a vessel (especially critical around spine or highly vascular areas). Then inject slowly; patient will often feel pressure or mild burning (from the anaesthetic). If using US, you can see the solution filling the target space.

After injection, the patient is usually observed briefly (15–30 minutes) to ensure no immediate reaction (like an allergic reaction or acute numbness/weakness if a nerve was affected by anaesthetic). They may experience immediate relief from the lidocaine—often a welcome "wow, the pain is gone!" moment that confirms diagnosis. This wears off in a few hours, and there may be a transient post-injection flare (steroid flare) where pain worsens for a day due to crystal-induced irritation [30]. Advise patient to ice if needed and that this typically passes in 1–2 days. The steroid's effect usually starts within 24–48 hours and peaks around 1 week.

Post-injection, advise relative rest of that area for ~48 hours to let steroid exert anti-inflammatory effect without immediate overload (e.g. no heavy lifting with that limb, or if knee injection, minimise impact activities for a day or two). After that, gradually resume activity and especially take advantage of pain relief to engage in exercises. For example, after a subacromial injection, the shoulder pain might be much less, therefore after a brief period of relative rest, starting guided physiotherapy exercises can help improve range and strengthen without pain limiting it.

Potential Risks and Side Effects [33]

- *Localised side effects* [34]: Skin depigmentation or subcutaneous fat atrophy at the injection site is possible if steroid is deposited too superficially. This is seen especially in injections near the dermis (like superficial trigger finger injections or lateral epicondyle)—leaving a white patch or slight dent months later.
- *Tendon rupture:* Steroids can weaken collagen and inhibit tenocyte function transiently [35]. If injected directly into a tendon or given repeatedly around a tendon, there is a risk of tendon degeneration or rupture. Achilles tendon is notorious—steroid injections for Achilles tendinopathy are generally avoided or done with great caution under imaging to ensure not intratendinous.
- *Joint infection:* Septic arthritis or localised abscess is a rare but serious risk (estimated roughly 1 in 3000 to 1 in 15,000 for joint injections) [34]. Strict aseptic technique (including appropriate skin antisepsis and local infection-control precautions) reduces risk. Also, if a patient has infection elsewhere or is very immunosuppressed, might avoid injection or postpone. If a patient develops intense pain and fever after an injection beyond 24–48 h, they must be evaluated for infection.
- *Post-injection flare:* As mentioned, about 2–10% get a steroid flare—increased pain for a day or two [34]. It is usually managed with rest, ice and maybe a short course of NSAIDs or analgesic.

- *Facial flushing:* A curious benign side effect where some patients (especially women) develop flushing or redness of face within 1–2 days after a steroid injection, lasting ~1 day [34]. It is transient and not dangerous, but good to warn them so they are not alarmed.
- *Hyperglycaemia:* In diabetic patients, a spike in blood sugar can occur for a week or so after a steroid shot, especially with larger joint injections. This is because some steroid enters systemic circulation. Advise diabetic patients to monitor glucose closely for the next 1–2 weeks and adjust meds in consultation with their diabetic care provider if needed.
- *HPA axis suppression* [33]: Unlikely from a single injection, but if multiple large-dose injections are given, a small systemic absorption can in theory cause temporary adrenal suppression or affect other cortisol-related functions. Generally this is not an issue unless doing very frequent injections or in a very small patient.
- *Bleeding/bruising* [33]: If a patient is on anticoagulation, there is a small risk of bleeding or haematoma at the injection site. Current thinking is injections can still be done on anticoagulated patients (e.g. on warfarin with INR in therapeutic range) with a fine needle and good technique, but perhaps avoid deep spinal injections under high anticoagulation due to catastrophic risks. For patients taking anticoagulants, bleeding risk should be considered according to the injection site, drug, renal function and local guidance; interruption is usually unnecessary for many peripheral injections but may be required for higher-risk deep or spinal procedures.
- *Allergy* [33]: True allergy to injected steroids or lidocaine is rare. Most "allergies" are either vasovagal reactions or anxiety. But if someone has a confirmed lidocaine allergy, one can do the injection with saline or just steroid alone (though that will hurt more). If they have had an allergic reaction to one form of steroid (some are compounded with certain preservatives), switch to a different preparation.

Non-corticosteroid Injections

- *Platelet-rich plasma (PRP)* [28]: Involves drawing the patient's blood, concentrating platelets and injecting into the injured tissue (commonly used in chronic tendinopathies such as tennis elbow/lateral elbow tendinopathy, and mild knee OA). The platelets release growth factors that might stimulate healing. Evidence for PRP is variable: some RCTs show benefit in lateral epicondylitis and knee OA compared to steroid (particularly longer term); others are inconclusive. It is generally safe (using patient's own blood), but it is costly and not universally available.
- *Prolotherapy* [36]: Injection of an irritant solution (like dextrose) to intentionally cause a localised inflammation and promote connective tissue strengthening. Used in ligament laxity or tendinopathies. Mixed evidence, but some patients respond. Multiple sessions are usually needed.
- *Hyaluronic acid (viscosupplementation)* [37]: Mainly for knee OA, not soft tissue per se. It is a series of injections intended to modify the viscoelastic properties of synovial fluid and potentially reduce pain in knee osteoarthritis, though evidence is mixed.

- *Botulinum toxin* [38]: In some refractory focal muscle spasm pain or conditions like refractory tennis elbow, there have been trials injecting Botox to relieve muscle overactivity.

In conclusion, injection therapy, particularly with corticosteroids, can be a powerful intervention for soft tissue rheumatic conditions. Its role is often to provide rapid symptom relief and anti-inflammatory effect, which can then be leveraged by the patient to engage in rehabilitative exercises more effectively. It is rarely a standalone cure (except in a few scenarios); rather, it is one component of the multidisciplinary approach. Proper patient selection, technique (with imaging guidance when indicated) and post-injection management maximise benefits and minimise risks.

The clinician should always ensure that the indication is solid (e.g. you confirm via exam or imaging that the trochanteric bursa is the pain source before injecting it) and that the patient understands the injection is to reduce pain and inflammation but that they will still need to do the follow-up exercises or therapy to address underlying issues.

When to Refer to Orthopaedics, Pain Specialists or MSK Radiology

While many musculoskeletal soft tissue problems can be managed non-surgically by rheumatologists, physiatrists or primary care, there are situations where specialist referral is prudent. Knowing those thresholds ensures patients receive advanced care when needed and prevents prolonged suffering or permanent deficits.

Referral to Orthopaedic Surgery

Orthopaedic surgeons specialise in operative management of musculoskeletal issues. Indications to refer a soft tissue condition to an orthopaedic (or sports medicine orthopaedist) include the following:

- *Failure of conservative treatment:* A patient with a tendinopathy or bursitis that has not responded to comprehensive conservative measures (rest, therapy, injections) over a reasonable time (usually 6 months or more) may be considered for surgical evaluation. For example, lateral epicondylitis unresponsive to >6–12 months of therapy and injections could be evaluated for surgical release/debridement.
- *Complete tears or severe structural lesions:* If imaging or exam reveals a complete tear of a tendon that is unlikely to heal on its own, early surgical referral is indicated. For instance, a young athlete with an acute full-thickness rotator cuff tear or Achilles tendon rupture should see orthopaedics promptly because surgical repair within weeks yields the best outcomes. Similarly, complete tear of the anterior cruciate ligament in a young patient often requires reconstruction for stability if they wish to return to cutting/pivoting sports.
- *Progressive weakness or loss of function:* If a soft tissue issue is causing neurological compromise or significant functional decline. For example, a large disc

herniation compressing a nerve root causing muscle weakness (foot drop) or a carpal tunnel syndrome causing thenar muscle atrophy—these may necessitate surgical decompression sooner rather than later.

- *Suspicion of neoplasm or unusual pathology:* If imaging or clinical picture is atypical and suggests a possibility of a tumour (e.g. a soft tissue mass or a non-resolving "tendinitis" with night pain and systemic symptoms), an orthopaedic oncologist referral for biopsy may be needed. Fortunately rare, but one must be vigilant.
- *Mechanical locking or instability:* If a joint or structure has mechanical issues like a loose body causing locking (e.g. pieces of cartilage in the knee locking motion or a flap tear of the glenoid labrum causing shoulder catching), surgical intervention to remove or repair is often indicated. In soft tissue context, a snapping scapula due to a bony spur could be an example where surgery might be considered if conservative measures fail.
- *Refractory entrapment neuropathies:* Carpal tunnel syndrome or cubital tunnel syndrome that does not respond to splinting and injections (and especially if there is electrodiagnostic evidence of severe entrapment) should be referred for release surgery to prevent permanent nerve damage.
- *Advanced osteoarthritis or degenerative conditions:* Not exactly "soft tissue" but often comanaged by rheumatologists. If a patient's joint osteoarthritis is severe on imaging and pain is debilitating despite conservative management (analgesia, physiotherapy, injections), refer to orthopaedics for consideration of joint replacement (hip, knee) or other surgeries (e.g. shoulder replacement). This is usually after exhausting other options or if patient is ready for a definitive solution.

When referring to orthopaedics, ensure the patient is medically optimised for potential surgery (like addressing uncontrolled diabetes or smoking cessation, as those affect healing). Also set patient expectations: discuss potential surgical outcomes vs risks, so they are mentally prepared and can ask the surgeon informed questions.

Referral to Pain Specialists (Pain Management Clinics)

Pain specialists focus on advanced pain control, including interventional procedures and multidisciplinary pain rehabilitation. Consider referral when:

- *Chronic pain with multifactorial elements:* If a patient's pain has become chronic and diffuse (like a fibromyalgia patient with severe disabling pain or chronic low back pain with psychological overlay) and is not improving with standard interventions, a pain clinic can provide more intensive multidisciplinary programmes (pain psychology, biofeedback, coping strategies) or medication management of more complex regimens.
- *Need for advanced analgesic techniques:* For example, epidural steroid injections for radiculopathy, facet joint injections or radiofrequency ablation for facet-mediated back pain and sympathetic nerve blocks for CRPS (complex regional pain syndrome). These are typically done by pain specialists under

fluoroscopic or CT guidance. If a patient has a pain condition that could benefit from these procedures, referral is indicated. For example, a herniated lumbar disc with persistent sciatica—consider an epidural injection by a pain specialist if not improving.

- *Consideration of neuromodulation:* If a patient has refractory neuropathic pain or CRPS, pain specialists might evaluate for spinal cord stimulation or intrathecal pain pump as options. This is usually after failure of conservative and less invasive measures.
- *Chronic opioid management:* Rheumatologists generally try to avoid long-term opioids for nonmalignant pain, but if a patient has ended up on high-dose opioids or requires opioid rotation/tapering or careful monitoring, a pain management specialist may take over that aspect. They can also explore alternatives (like methadone or buprenorphine or multimodal analgesia) in complex cases.
- *Procedures like trigger point injections or Botox:* If needed extensively or in areas the rheumatologist is not comfortable injecting, pain clinics often do trigger point injections in multiple areas, Botox for myofascial pain, etc.
- *Chronic headaches or fibromyalgia overlaps:* Some pain clinics have programmes for chronic headaches (nerve blocks, Botox for migraine) or fibromyalgia (they might coordinate therapy, meds, etc., often overlapping with what rheum does, but in some systems, pain clinics take fibromyalgia patients to manage).
- *Patient needing structured pain rehabilitation programme:* Some pain centres have 2–4-week outpatient programmes where a patient attends daily sessions of physiotherapy, occupational therapy, group therapy, etc. A fibromyalgia patient with severe dysfunction might benefit from such a comprehensive programme—referral to pain rehabilitation programme is warranted if available.

Pain specialists often work closely with psychologists and physiotherapy, offering a truly interdisciplinary approach. It is especially useful when pain is disproportionate to objective findings or accompanied by significant psychosocial issues—they address the whole picture.

Referral to Musculoskeletal Radiology (Interventional Radiology or MSK Radiologist)

MSK radiologists can perform specialised image-guided interventions and diagnostic imaging beyond what a standard clinic can do. Scenarios for referral:

- *Deep or complex injection needs:* If a rheumatologist or sports medicine consultant needs a difficult injection done with imaging and they themselves do not perform it, an MSK radiologist can. For instance, a sacroiliac joint injection under fluoroscopy or CT, a piriformis muscle injection for piriformis syndrome or an injection around a nerve (like stellate ganglion block for CRPS, though often pain docs do that too). Also, injections like barbotage of a calcific tendon (using a needle under US to aspirate calcium deposits) can be done by MSK radiologists.

- *Diagnostic imaging consultation:* If initial imaging is inconclusive or if an MRI/US shows something unclear, an MSK radiologist's opinion can be sought. They can also perform MR arthrograms (inject contrast into a joint to better visualise labral tears or subtle rotator cuff tears).
- *Biopsy of soft tissue lesions:* If there is a suspicious mass or atypical swelling, an MSK radiologist can often do a needle biopsy under imaging guidance (US or CT) to get a tissue diagnosis without open surgery.
- *Advanced procedures:* Things like radiofrequency ablation of certain nerve branches (pain docs or radiologists do this for facet joint pain or for calcaneal spur pain by ablating a nerve), cement augmentation (vertebroplasty for compression fractures), etc. often involve interventional radiology.

Referral to Sport and Exercise Medicine Physicians
This is another category—sport and exercise medicine consultants often do many of the things we have mentioned: injections, coordinated rehabilitation and prescribed therapies. If available, they can take on non-surgical MSK cases that are complex. For example, a patient with chronic back pain and previous spinal surgery might be comanaged with a sports medicine physician who focuses on functional improvement, brace prescriptions, etc. In some healthcare settings, fibromyalgia or chronic pain management might be shared with a pain clinic.

Coordination of Care
Often, the patient's case might involve multiple specialists sequentially or concurrently. For example, a patient with knee osteoarthritis and chronic back pain might see rheumatology for overall plan, ortho for a knee injection or replacement, pain clinic for an epidural injection and physiotherapy throughout. Good communication and clear delineation of roles helps avoid confusion (for instance, ensuring multiple steroid injections are not given too close together by different docs or that medication regimens are coordinated).

Patient Factors in Referral Decisions
Always consider patient preference—some are very averse to surgery, so you might continue conservative measures longer, while others want a definitive fix and are eager for surgical opinion. Also consider timing—an athlete mid-season might be referred sooner for a surgical opinion to be ready for next season, whereas a non-athlete might be okay with waiting longer to see if rehabilitation works. Occupational needs are also a factor: if a manual labourer has a rotator cuff tear and cannot work, early surgical referral is more urgent than in a retiree who can manage with modifications.

Red Flag Referrals [39] Always keep in mind red flags that mandate urgent referral:

- Suspected septic arthritis or osteomyelitis
- Cauda equina syndrome signs in back pain

- Suspected compartment syndrome in an extremity
- Deep vein thrombosis suspected in a calf that was thought to be just muscle injury

In summary, referrals to orthopaedics are mainly for possible surgical interventions when conservative measures fail or when structural problems require fixing. Pain specialists come in when advanced pain control or interventions are needed beyond the standard scope of practice, and MSK radiologists assist in specialised diagnostic or guided therapeutic procedures. Knowing when to escalate care to these specialists ensures patients do not endure prolonged ineffective treatment or risk permanent impairment. Conversely, avoiding premature referral for cases that can be managed non-surgically spares patients unnecessary invasive procedures.

Key Point It is often said in musculoskeletal care: *surgery should be the last option except when it should be the first.* In other words, most soft tissue issues resolve with rehabilitation (last option), except those few where surgery is clearly indicated early (first), like complete tendon ruptures or severe compressive neuropathies. Balancing that wisdom comes with clinical experience and careful patient evaluation.

Prevention and Recurrence Strategies

Preventing recurrence of musculoskeletal soft tissue problems is a crucial component of long-term management. Many conditions, once resolved, have a tendency to come back if predisposing factors remain unaddressed. Additionally, some chronic conditions can flare episodically (like chronic low back pain or tendinitis). Below are strategies to mitigate recurrence and maintain musculoskeletal health:

1. *Address Underlying Predisposing Factors:*
   - *Ergonomics* [4]: For work-related or posture-related issues, a thorough ergonomics assessment is key. For example, a person who developed cervical radiculopathy or trapezius myofascial pain from prolonged computer work should adjust monitor height (top of screen at eye level), use a document holder to avoid constant neck flexion, ensure supportive chair with armrests, etc. Similarly, a factory worker with repetitive wrist flexion tasks might need a modified tool or rotation of tasks to prevent reinjury of wrist tendons.
   - *Technique in sports:* Athletes should have their form evaluated by coaches or therapists. A runner with recurring shin splints may need gait analysis—sometimes a slight change in running form or cadence can reduce tibial stress. A tennis player with lateral epicondylitis may benefit from adjusting racket grip size or string tension and improving backhand technique to reduce strain on the elbow. Pitchers with shoulder/elbow issues often undergo biomechanical analysis to correct any unsafe throwing mechanics.
   - *Footwear and orthotics:* Many lower extremity issues (plantar fasciitis, Achilles tendinopathy, knee stress) can be aggravated by poor footwear or foot biomechanics [40]. Ensuring proper shoes for the activity (cushioned

running shoes replaced every ~500 miles, supportive shoes for standing work, etc.) is baseline. Custom or off-the-shelf orthotics may help those with flat feet or high arches to distribute forces evenly. For example, in plantar fasciitis, an orthotic with good arch support can take strain off the fascia and prevent recurrence.

- *Muscle imbalance correction:* Often one muscle group being much stronger/tighter than its opposing group leads to problems (e.g. quads vs hamstrings imbalance contributing to hamstring strains or patellofemoral pain). A balanced conditioning programme that strengthens the weaker and stretches the tighter muscles should continue even after initial rehabilitation. Patients should incorporate these into their regular exercise routine (like always doing hamstring strengthening if they are quad-dominant).
- *Weight management* [41]: Excess body weight increases stress on weight-bearing joints and tissues. Even a loss of 5–10% body weight can substantially reduce forces through the knees, feet and lower back. For chronic knee pain, weight loss is one of the most effective ways to lessen pain and improve function. Similarly, obesity is associated with tendinopathies (due to systemic inflammation and mechanical load). Encouraging and supporting weight loss through diet and exercise is critical in prevention of recurrence for many patients.
- *Bone health* [42]: For stress fractures or osteoporotic fractures, ensure underlying bone health is optimised. Adequate calcium/vitamin D, treating osteoporosis with medications if present and not overtraining in susceptible individuals (like female athlete triad cases) will prevent recurrences of bony injuries which often present as soft tissue pain initially.

2. *Ongoing Exercise and Conditioning* [43]

   "Graduation" from formal physiotherapy does not mean stop exercising. Patients should continue a maintenance exercise programme indefinitely:

   - *Stretching routine:* Keep doing daily or thrice weekly stretches for previously problematic areas. For example, someone with previous IT band syndrome should regularly stretch hip abductors and foam roll the IT band region, especially after exercise.
   - *Strength maintenance:* At least 2 days a week of strength exercises focusing on vulnerable areas. For example, a person with prior back pain should maintain core exercises as part of their weekly regimen. A runner with prior Achilles issue should do calf strengthening and eccentric heel drops weekly even when pain-free.
   - *Gradual resumption of new activities:* If starting a new activity or sport, apply principles of gradual progression to avoid injury. For example, if a patient who recovered from knee pain wants to start hiking, advise them to start with short, easy hikes and build up distance and elevation over weeks; do not jump into a 10-mile mountain hike on day 1.

   - *Cross-training:* Doing a variety of activities can prevent overuse from any single one. If someone recovered from a stress injury from running, incorporate cycling or swimming on alternate days to limit weekly impact mileage.
3. *Listen to early warning signs:* Educate patients to pay attention to mild symptoms—these are often signals to adjust behaviour before a full flare:
   - For instance, a slight twinge of familiar pain should prompt them to scale back activity a bit; do more stretching/icing that evening, rather than pushing through until it becomes severe. Many recurrent injuries happen because people ignore low-grade symptoms until they worsen.
   - Encourage the concept of "active rest"—if something starts hurting, reduce intensity or switch activities (e.g. do low-impact cardio instead of running for a few days) to allow recovery without complete inactivity.
4. *Periodic tune-ups:* Some patients benefit from periodic check-ins with a physiotherapist or trainer:
   - If they have a chronic condition like fibromyalgia or chronic back pain, maybe a physiotherapy session every few months to review their exercise programme, progress it and correct any form issues.
   - Those with heavy training schedules might see a sports physiotherapist or massage therapist for maintenance work (like an athlete getting regular sports massage or flexibility sessions to prevent soft tissue injuries).
   - If work tasks change or new equipment is introduced, an ergonomic reevaluation by occupational health can prevent new problems.
5. *Workplace and Lifestyle Adjustments for Sustainability:*
   - Suggest microbreaks for those in static postures (e.g. stand up and stretch every 30 minutes at a desk; during long drives, take a break every 1–2 hours to walk).
   - If someone's job is extremely physical, explore options for rotating tasks or using assistive devices (like hoists for heavy lifting and ergonomic tools) to reduce repetitive strain.
   - Emphasise general health: good sleep, stress management, avoiding smoking (smoking impairs tissue healing and is associated with back pain and poor disc health) and proper nutrition (for muscle recovery). These systemic factors affect recurrence risk.
6. *Support and Education*

   People who understand their condition and how to manage it are less likely to have recurrences or more likely to nip them early. Provide written home exercise instructions and links to reputable resources (like Arthritis Foundation or sports medicine websites for specific injuries). If a patient has an identified risk factor (e.g. hypermobility), ensure they know how to manage it lifelong (like protecting hypermobile joints with exercise and not overstretching already lax joints).

7. *Protective Gear* [44]

   In some cases, the continued use of protective gear can prevent recurrences:
   - Bracing: For example, an athlete with chronic ankle sprains might wear an ankle brace or tape during high-risk activities indefinitely. A weightlifter with a history of back injury might use a lifting belt for heavy lifts (though also needs core training).
   - Shoe insoles or proper footwear as mentioned—maybe a patient with history of metatarsalgia uses metatarsal pads in all their shoes going forward.
   - Splints at night: People with carpal tunnel might wear a wrist splint at night even after symptoms improve, to keep wrists neutral and avoid recurrence of nerve compression during sleep.

8. *Balancing Activity and Rest*

Overuse injuries often stem from doing too much too soon (as discussed). Encouraging patients to incorporate rest days in their routines is important. Athletes often follow periodisation with built-in rest or lighter weeks after heavy training blocks. Nonathletes also should avoid consistently pushing themselves without respite. Also, vary tasks (do not hammer or type all day without variation—mix in other duties if possible).

9. *Maintenance of Healthy Habits*

For conditions like fibromyalgia, recurrence of flares can be minimised by maintaining a healthy baseline routine: regular exercise, pacing activities, continuing any helpful practices (yoga, meditation, etc.) and promptly addressing minor stressors or mood dips (like resuming therapy if needed). The chronic nature of such conditions means ongoing self-care is essential to keep symptoms at bay.

10. *Follow-Up Monitoring*

For certain injuries, schedule a follow-up (even by phone or email) some months down the line to see if patient maintained improvements. Sometimes that check-in prompts them to stick with exercises if they have been slacking.

In essence, prevention of recurrence involves embedding the gains of therapy into the patient's lifestyle permanently. The episodic care model (treat then forget) often fails because as soon as pain is gone, people revert to old habits. By instilling the notion that they have a chronic vulnerability that needs minding (not in a fearful way but in a proactive way), patients can take ownership of prevention.

An analogy often given to patients: "Your exercises and ergonomic changes are like brushing your teeth – you have to keep doing them to prevent problems, not just do them until the cavity is filled". Another: "Think of your problematic body part as having a 'maintenance required' light – you need to keep up the maintenance to keep it running smoothly".

Finally, sometimes despite best efforts, recurrences happen. Have a plan for early intervention if they do (e.g. they know to start their exercise routine more intensely or come back for a booster physiotherapy session or get a timely injection if needed). Quick action can make a recurrence just a blip rather than a full regression.

Building a Patient-Centred Management Plan [45]

A patient-centred management plan means that the patient's individual goals, preferences and circumstances are at the core of the strategy. It also implies shared decision-making—the clinician and patient collaborate as partners. Here is how to build such a plan:

1. *Solicit the Patient's Goals and Expectations*

Start by asking open-ended questions: "What are you most hoping to achieve from treatment? What activities do you miss doing that you'd like to get back to? What are your biggest concerns or fears about your condition?" The answers might reveal, for example, that a grandmother with knee pain values being able to play on the floor with her grandkids more than being able to run a 5 K (so focus on functional mobility, not running endurance). Or a young office worker with back pain might say he is afraid of ending up like his father who had multiple surgeries—so his goal is to manage this conservatively and avoid surgery. By understanding these, you can tailor your approach and also manage expectations. If someone expects a complete cure in 1 week from a long-standing condition, gentle education is needed to set realistic timelines.

2. *Incorporate Patient Preferences in Treatment Modalities*

Some patients might have strong preferences or aversions. One patient might say, "I really do not want injections"—then you emphasise other pathways and only consider injections if absolutely necessary or if they later become open to it. Another might say, "I prefer natural or active treatments over taking medications"—then you focus heavily on therapy, exercise and maybe supplements, using meds minimally. If a patient hates going to the gym but loves gardening, your exercise plan might revolve around activities they enjoy or home-based routines rather than insisting on a gym programme, thereby improving adherence. Cultural preferences also matter; for example, some cultures value massage or heat therapy—you can integrate those if it helps engagement (even if just as adjunct). The plan should also respect religious or spiritual practices (like scheduling around prayer times or using mind-body approaches if they are open to them).

3. *Education and Health Literacy*
   A patient-centred plan ensures the patient understands their condition and the reasoning behind each part of the plan. Use lay language, visuals (diagrams of

their anatomy or exercises) and analogies that resonate with the patient's life (e.g. if the patient is an engineer, you might use an analogy of "mechanical stress and strain" to explain tendon overload). Check their understanding by asking them to summarise what the plan is ("Just to be sure we're on the same page, can you tell me how you'll manage your back pain this week?"). This helps identify any confusion or concerns.

- If a patient has low health literacy or a language barrier, use teach-back method, provide brochures in their language or enlist help of interpreters/family. A plan that the patient does not truly comprehend is not patient-centred.

4. *Shared Decision-Making* [46]

Present options with their pros and cons, and involve the patient in choosing. For instance, for knee osteoarthritis, you might outline: weight loss, physiotherapy, NSAIDs, steroid injection, hyaluronic injection and surgery. Discuss each in context of their condition (e.g. "Given your X-rays are moderate and you're 50, we have multiple options. How do you feel about injections? Some patients prefer to try an injection to see if it helps before considering surgery. Others want to avoid needles and try other things first. Let's discuss what you're leaning towards".). This invites the patient's values. For more complex decisions (like whether to have a surgery or not), tools like decision aids (pamphlets or videos explaining options) can help. It is also okay to give a recommendation based on expertise but still honour patient's choice (e.g. "Medically, I'd recommend we attempt at least 3 months of therapy before thinking of surgery. Does that align with your own goals?").

5. *Multidisciplinary Coordination with Patient at the Centre*

If multiple providers are involved, ensure the patient is not lost between them. Provide a written plan (or at least a summary) that the patient can share with others. Encourage the patient to keep a folder with their exercise handouts, appointment notes, etc. If the patient consents, you can directly communicate with the physiotherapist or other team members to unify the plan.

6. *Flexibility and Patient Autonomy*

A patient-centred plan should be flexible to adjust as the patient's situation evolves. Maybe the patient's work schedule changes, and they cannot do morning physiotherapy sessions—find an alternative (evening class or home programme). Or if one approach is not working for them (they tried pool therapy and disliked it), pivot to something else (maybe stationary bike or Tai Chi). The plan is not a rigid prescription; it is a living plan that can be reformulated with patient input at each step.

7. *Empowerment and Self-Efficacy*

One of the ultimate goals is to increase the patient's confidence in managing their condition. This means gradually shifting responsibility to them in a supportive way. For instance, instead of "the therapist will fix you", frame it as "the therapist will teach you how to fix yourself and be your coach". Celebrate successes—"You improved your shoulder range by 20 degrees, that's your hard work paying off!"—which reinforces their role in improvement. Encourage self-monitoring (like a pain/activity diary) if they are willing, which makes them an active participant. When they have setbacks, involve them in problem-solving: "What do you think made your knee worse last week? What can we adjust together"?

8. *Psychosocial Considerations* [47]

A truly patient-centred plan considers stressors, mental health and support systems. If a patient is a caregiver for someone else, their ability to do exercises or attend appointments might be limited—maybe arrange home physiotherapy or provide more home-based instructions. If depression or anxiety is present, incorporate treatment for those (perhaps referral to counselling) into the plan, as it will affect outcomes.

9. *Accessibility*

Ensure the plan is realistic given the patient's resources. For example, do not prescribe aquatic therapy if they have no pool access or cannot swim. If language is a barrier, ensure translators or multilingual providers are engaged.

10. *Follow-Up and Feedback Loop*

Let the patient know that the plan is not set in stone and that their feedback is crucial. Schedule follow-ups to check progress, and explicitly ask at follow-up, "How do you feel the plan is working for you? What challenges are you facing in following it?" If something is not working (maybe they hate a medication's side effects or find an exercise too painful), immediately validate their concern and adjust. This shows respect for their experience and that the plan is a collaboration.

By implementing all the above, the resulting management plan should feel to the patient like it is their plan (not just the doctor's orders). That ownership increases adherence and satisfaction. It often leads to better outcomes because the interventions chosen are more likely to fit into the patient's life.

Patient-centred care has been associated with improved outcomes in many studies (like better pain control and functional improvements), likely because when patients are engaged and agree with the plan, they follow through more consistently. It also improves the therapeutic relationship, which itself can positively influence results (through better communication, trust and placebo/healing effects of feeling cared for).

Red Flags and Pitfalls in Treatment [39]

Not every musculoskeletal pain is benign, and not every treatment approach works as intended. It is critical to remain vigilant for "red flags"—signs or symptoms that suggest a potentially serious underlying condition or an alternative diagnosis that should not be managed with routine conservative care. Additionally, certain pitfalls in treatment can hinder recovery or even harm the patient. We will outline these to ensure safe practice and optimal outcomes.

Red Flags in Musculoskeletal Pain [39]

These are warning signs that something more ominous than a simple soft tissue injury might be present. If any of these are noted, further investigation (imaging, labs) and possibly specialist referral (e.g. to oncology, spine surgeon, etc.) are warranted:

- *Constitutional symptoms:* Unexplained weight loss, fevers or chills accompanying musculoskeletal pain raise concern for infection or malignancy. For example, a patient with chronic back pain who has lost 10 kg in 2 months without trying should be evaluated for possible spinal tumour or systemic illness.
- *Night pain and rest pain:* Pain that wakes the patient from sleep consistently, or is present at rest and not relieved by any changes in position, is a red flag. Soft tissue rheum pains like tendinitis usually ease with rest. Persistent night pain might indicate a tumour (bone cancer often hurts more at night) or infection.
- *Neurological deficits:* Significant weakness, loss of sensation in a dermatomal pattern and loss of bowel/bladder control are red flags for neural compromise. For instance, foot drop in the context of back pain may indicate a large disc herniation compressing L5 nerve root or even a central lesion like a tumour. Cauda equina syndrome (from a massive disc or tumour compressing cauda equina) presents with saddle anaesthesia, bilateral leg weakness and incontinence—a surgical emergency [48].
- *Significant trauma or fracture risk:* A history of major trauma (like a fall from height or car accident) preceding pain should prompt a search for fractures or internal injuries, not just assume a sprain. In older patients or those with osteoporosis, even minor trauma can cause fractures (like a vertebral compression fracture causing back pain after just a sneeze or stepping off a curb).
- *Swollen joint or erythema beyond typical:* If a patient presents with a very hot, red, swollen joint (especially with fever), think septic arthritis or crystalline arthritis (gout). A very red, warm area in soft tissue could be cellulitis or abscess, not just bursitis. For example, what might be presumed "olecranon bursitis" if very red and tender might actually be infected bursitis—aspiration and analysis needed rather than immediate steroid injection.
- *Claudication or circulatory compromise:* Leg pain that occurs with walking and is relieved by rest might be vascular claudication (peripheral artery disease) rather than just muscle strain. Similarly, if an extremity is pale and pulseless or has differences in temperature, consider vascular issues (like thoracic outlet

syndrome compressing subclavian artery in an arm causing exertional pain or critical limb ischemia in legs).
- *History of cancer or immunosuppression:* A patient with a past cancer who has new bone pain must be evaluated for metastasis. Immunosuppressed patients (e.g. on biologics or diabetics) with back pain could have unusual infections (like vertebral osteomyelitis or epidural abscess) that present subtly but need urgent care (clues may be mild fever, high ESR/CRP or just persistent pain unrelieved by rest or position).
- *Atypical age or location:* Low back pain in a 20-year-old male with stiffness might hint at axial spondyloarthritis (inflammatory back pain)—consider inflammatory markers and imaging. Lateral hip pain in a young child might be Legg-Calve-Perthes or a slipped capital femoral epiphysis rather than trochanteric bursitis. Know typical age ranges: for example, older patient with new unilateral shoulder pain could be a rotator cuff tear or polymyalgia rheumatica (especially if bilateral with stiffness and high ESR).
- *Multiple joint involvement or systemic signs:* If what was thought a localised problem starts involving multiple sites (like symmetric hand joint pains and morning stiffness systemic upset), consider an underlying inflammatory disease (like rheumatoid arthritis) rather than separate soft tissue issues. Similarly, connective tissue diseases might present with diffuse pain plus rashes or Raynaud's—need workup and not just physiotherapy for pain.

In presence of red flags, typical conservative management should be paused and appropriate diagnostic work-up done (like imaging, X-ray, MRI, lab tests: ESR, CRP, FBC, etc., and referrals as needed).

Pitfalls in Treatment

These are common mistakes or oversights that can impede recovery or harm the patient:

- *Overreliance on passive modalities:* Some patients (and clinicians) fall into the trap of repeatedly using passive treatments (like endless heat, ultrasound and massage) without moving on to active rehabilitation. While those modalities can help short term, they will not address underlying weaknesses or biomechanical issues. Pitfall: The patient feels temporarily better but does not build strength or endurance, so the problem returns as soon as they resume normal activities. It is important to transition to exercise and self-management.
- *Ignoring the psychological aspect:* Dismissing the psychosocial contributors (stress, mood, fear-avoidance) can derail recovery. For example, a patient with chronic low back pain who is terrified of reinjury might not engage properly in exercises unless the fear is addressed. Pitfall: the provider keeps increasing physiotherapy intensity, but the patient unconsciously guards or avoids, limiting progress. Or the patient might have secondary gain issues (like compensation) that need to be delicately managed. Not addressing these can result in chronic disability.

- *Inappropriate use of steroids or NSAIDs:* While these are helpful, misuse can cause issues. Pitfalls include giving too many steroid injections too frequently (leading to tissue damage or systemic effects) [33] or injecting into an incorrect diagnosis (e.g. injecting what is thought to be "inflammation" when it is actually a partial tendon tear or infection, which steroids would worsen) [33]. Similarly, long-term high-dose NSAIDs without considering gastroprotection or patient risk factors can cause ulcers or kidney issues. Always review medication plan for safety given patient's comorbidities.
- *Skimping on patient education:* If a patient does not understand their condition or treatment rationale, they might be nonadherent. For instance, not explaining that an exercise might initially cause some soreness can lead a patient to abandon it thinking it is harmful. Or not explaining the expected timeline—patient might quit physiotherapy after two sessions because they are not cured (thinking it should be immediate). It is a pitfall if we do not set expectations (like "usually it takes 4–6 weeks of regular exercise to see significant improvement").
- *Poor technique or form in exercises* [49]*:* If patients do exercises incorrectly at home (say, a squat with knees caving in, causing more knee pain, or a rotator cuff exercise using upper trap compensation), they may hurt themselves or not benefit. It is a pitfall not to check form or to prescribe too advanced exercises without adequate supervision/training. Solution: have physiotherapist or trained person teach them properly, maybe provide video links or written details and follow up on their form.
- *Failure to recognise when to escalate or refer:* Sometimes clinicians or patients persist with conservative management for too long when it is clear it is not working. Pitfall: a patient with a large rotator cuff tear doing physiotherapy for a year with no improvement in strength—muscle might be atrophying and tendon retracting, making eventual surgical repair harder. Knowing the window of opportunity is important. Similarly, not referring a nerve compression in time could lead to permanent nerve damage that could have been prevented by timely surgery. Always reassess every few weeks—if a reasonable plateau or worsening, consider imaging or referral
- *Neglecting whole patient:* A pitfall is to focus only on the painful area and ignore related factors. Example: treating Achilles tendinopathy but ignoring very tight hamstrings and weak glutes that are altering gait—the Achilles keeps getting overloaded due to these issues, so the problem recurs. Or treating one knee's arthritis and forgetting to check the other leg which might be overworked—soon the other knee flares. A holistic view is needed to avoid chasing one site after another.
- *Inadequate follow-up:* Not scheduling follow-up after an intervention monitor outcome is a pitfall. The patient may drift, either not improving and feeling lost, or even worsen. Timely follow-up allows modifications to plan and catches complications (e.g. if you perform an injection, follow up to ensure it helped and no problems).

- *Poor communication among providers:* If multiple providers are involved and they do not communicate, the plan can become fragmented or even conflicting. Coordination is key to avoid this pitfall.
- *Prescribing opioids early or inappropriately:* Using strong pain medication as an easy fix can lead to dependence or mask underlying issues. For instance, giving opioids for chronic back pain without addressing core strengthening—patient feels somewhat better, avoids exercise because pain is dulled and then becomes tolerant to opioids and still has weak back. Now there are two problems: chronic pain and opioid dependence. The pitfall is not utilising safer modalities first and educating patient on realistic pain management.
- *Not considering patient's life context:* A plan might fail because it did not fit the patient's lifestyle (e.g. daily exercises for a single mother of three with no spare time—she does not do them). Pitfall is blaming patient for non-compliance when the plan was impractical. We should tailor to what is doable for them (maybe shorter exercise bouts or integrating with daily tasks).
- *Rushing the rehabilitation:* Advancing too quickly can reinjure. For example, an athlete feels a bit better and the therapist or coach pushes them back to full sport too soon, causing relapse. This pitfall often comes from external pressures (the athlete's desire or team's push). Need to ensure objective criteria are met before full return.
- *Applying one-size-fits-all protocols:* Each patient is different. A pitfall is rigidly adhering to a protocol even when patient is not responding or has unique factors. Example: typical protocol says 6 weeks of physiotherapy but patient clearly plateaued at 3 weeks—continuing the same thing three more weeks wasted time. Or typical exercise is painful for that patient due to a variant anatomy—but we keep insisting because "protocol says so". Better to adjust to patient.
- *Overlooking comorbid conditions:* Sometimes, a patient's other health issues affect MSK treatment but are ignored. For example, uncontrolled diabetes can impair healing of a tendon or increase risk in injection. Osteoporosis if not addressed can cause repeated fractures. Depression if untreated can foil efforts as patient may lack motivation. Holistic care means managing those concurrently or liaising with their other doctors.

Recognising red flags early can literally be life-saving or prevent serious disability. Avoiding pitfalls requires experience, constant reevaluation and a humble attitude that if something is not working, reconsider the approach or diagnosis.

In practice, maintaining a checklist mindset helps: For any persistent or atypical case, mentally run through red flags (weight, fever, neuro exam, etc.). For management, periodically step back and ask, "Is the patient better? If not, why? Are we missing something? Is the execution of plan okay? Is the patient doing their part, if not, why"?

Encourage an environment where patients also feel comfortable voicing concerns ("The exercise you gave makes my pain worse"), so those pitfalls are identified instead of patient silently suffering or quitting.

Finally, continuous learning and collaboration can minimise pitfalls—for example, discussing tough cases in a multidisciplinary meeting can provide new insights or updating knowledge on guidelines (like knowing when imaging is indicated to catch red flags).

By being aware of these red flags and pitfalls, clinicians can navigate treatment more safely and effectively, ensuring serious conditions are not overlooked and that their rehabilitation efforts lead to steady, safe improvement rather than frustration or harm.

Key Learning Points

- Rehabilitation of soft tissue and musculoskeletal conditions is best approached with a multimodal strategy, combining patient education, exercise therapy, physical modalities and appropriate medical or interventional treatments. No single modality is a panacea; integrating multiple approaches yields optimal results.
- Physiotherapy principles include pain relief techniques (heat, cold, TENS, manual therapy) to allow movement and progressive restoration of mobility (stretching, joint mobilisations), followed by strengthening and stabilisation exercises to address muscle imbalances and support joints. Emphasis is placed on functional exercises that translate to everyday activities or sports-specific demands.
- Exercise prescription should be tailored to the individual using the FITT criteria—specifying type (aerobic, strengthening, flexibility, etc.), frequency, intensity and duration. Progression of exercise should be gradual (typically not more than ~10% increase per week) to avoid reinjury and guided by patient tolerance. Pacing and rest are crucial for chronic pain patients to prevent flare-ups.
- Injections are a valuable tool for conditions like bursitis, tenosynovitis and arthritic flares. They provide potent local anti-inflammatory effect and pain relief, facilitating rehabilitation. For example, subacromial steroid injections relieve shoulder impingement pain to improve ROM; de Quervain's tenosynovitis often resolves with a single sheath injection. Injections should be used judiciously—typically limited to a few times a year in a given site—to avoid side effects (e.g. tendon weakening or rupture, skin depigmentation).
- Ultrasound guidance improves injection accuracy and safety. It is particularly useful for deep or anatomically complex targets (e.g. guiding a steroid injection into a small joint or around a tendon while avoiding nerves/vessels) and has been shown to enhance outcomes in certain cases by ensuring the medication reaches the intended tissue.
- Preventing recurrence of soft tissue injuries is an integral part of management. This includes educating patients on ergonomics (e.g. proper workstation setup to avoid repetitive strain), encouraging ongoing exercise and stretching routines for maintenance and addressing risk factors like muscle imbalances or poor technique (with coaching or therapy) and lifestyle modifications (weight loss, appropriate footwear/orthotics, etc.) to reduce undue stress on tissues. Patients should learn to listen to early warning signs of overuse and intervene early (relative rest, icing, etc.) to avert full relapse.

- Patient-centred management involves aligning the treatment plan with the patient's goals, preferences and life context. Shared decision-making improves adherence—for instance, incorporating a patient's preferred exercise activities into their rehabilitation programme or negotiating treatment options (like trying physiotherapy before considering surgery if that is the patient's wish). Effective communication and education empower patients, making them active participants in their recovery.
- Red flags in musculoskeletal presentations (such as unexplained weight loss, night pain, neurological deficits, fevers or history of malignancy) should prompt further investigation rather than routine conservative treatment. These signs may indicate serious underlying conditions (infection, tumour, fracture, inflammatory disease) that require urgent or specific management beyond standard soft tissue rehabilitation.
- Common treatment pitfalls to avoid include overreliance on passive treatments without progressing to active rehabilitation, neglecting psychosocial factors (like fear of movement or depression) that impede recovery, poorly communicated or overly rigid treatment plans that do not fit the patient's lifestyle and missing timely referral for surgical opinion when indicated (leading to prolonged dysfunction). Regular reevaluation and flexibility in the management plan help circumvent these pitfalls.
- Rehabilitation is not a linear process—flare-ups can occur and should not be viewed as failures but as signals to adjust the plan. Teaching patients how to manage minor flares (e.g. temporarily reducing intensity, using modalities at home and then gradually ramping back up) is key for long-term self-management of chronic musculoskeletal conditions.
- Successful outcomes in soft tissue rheumatology are measured not just by pain reduction on a scale but by functional improvements and patient satisfaction—for example, the patient can return to playing with their children, resume their sport or work with less limitation. Always tie treatment goals to meaningful functional targets for the patient.

References

1. Wang F, Zhang Q-B, Zhou Y, Chen S, Huang P-P, Liu Y, et al. The mechanisms and treatments of muscular pathological changes in immobilization-induced joint contracture: a literature review. Chinese J Traumatol = Zhonghua chuang shang za zhi [Internet]. 2019;22(2):93–8. Available from: http://www.ncbi.nlm.nih.gov/pubmed/30928194.
2. Kannus P. Immobilization or early mobilization after an acute soft-tissue injury? Phys Sportsmed [Internet]. 2000;28(3):55–63. Available from: http://www.ncbi.nlm.nih.gov/pubmed/20086628.
3. Dubois B, Esculier J-F. Soft-tissue injuries simply need PEACE and LOVE. Br J Sports Med [Internet]. 2020;54(2):72–3. Available from: http://www.ncbi.nlm.nih.gov/pubmed/31377722.
4. Santos W, Rojas C, Isidoro R, Lorente A, Dias A, Mariscal G, et al. Efficacy of ergonomic interventions on work-related musculoskeletal pain: a systematic review and meta-analysis. J Clin Med [Internet]. 2025;14(9). Available from: http://www.ncbi.nlm.nih.gov/pubmed/40364066.

5. Machado AFP, Santana EF, Tacani PM, Liebano RE. The effects of transcutaneous electrical nerve stimulation on tissue repair: a literature review. Can J Plast Surg [Internet]. 2012;20(4):237–40. Available from: http://www.ncbi.nlm.nih.gov/pubmed/24294017.
6. Papadopoulos ES, Mani R. The role of ultrasound therapy in the management of musculoskeletal soft tissue pain. Int J Low Extrem Wounds [Internet]. 2020;19(4):350–8. Available from: http://www.ncbi.nlm.nih.gov/pubmed/32856521.
7. Jurecka A, Papież M, Skucińska P, Gądek A. Evaluating the effectiveness of soft tissue therapy in the treatment of disorders and postoperative conditions of the knee joint-a systematic review. J Clin Med [Internet]. 2021;10(24). Available from: http://www.ncbi.nlm.nih.gov/pubmed/34945240.
8. Berger AA, Liu Y, Nguyen J, Spraggins R, Reed DS, Lee C, et al. Efficacy of acupuncture in the treatment of fibromyalgia. Orthop Rev (Pavia) [Internet]. 2021;13(2):25085. Available from: http://www.ncbi.nlm.nih.gov/pubmed/34745475.
9. El-Khateeb YS, Mahmoud AG, Mohamed MH, Abd El-Azeim AS. Influence of adding strain-counterstrain to standard therapy on axioscapular muscles amplitude and fatigue in mechanical neck pain: a single-blind, randomized trial. Eur J Phys Rehabil Med [Internet]. 2022;58(4):621–9. Available from: http://www.ncbi.nlm.nih.gov/pubmed/35666489.
10. Sivan M, Bhakta B. Restoring mobility: theories, technologies and effective treatments. Clin Med [Internet]. 2008;8(6):596–600. Available from: http://www.ncbi.nlm.nih.gov/pubmed/19149281.
11. Shahzad A, Azhar M, Zafar H, Khan MA, Shakir S. Therapeutic effects of mobilization in alleviating pain and improving shoulder mobility in adhesive capsulitis—a systematic review. J Musculoskelet Surg Res [Internet]. 2024;8:97. Available from: https://www.journalmsr.com/therapeutic-effects-of-mobilization-in-alleviating-pain-and-improving-shoulder-mobility-in-adhesive-capsulitis-a-systematic-review/ .
12. Lu L, Robinson M, Tan Y, Goonewardena K, Guo X, Mareels I, et al. Effective assessments of a short-duration poor posture on upper limb muscle fatigue before physical exercise. Front Physiol [Internet]. 2020;11:541974. Available from: http://www.ncbi.nlm.nih.gov/pubmed/33132916.
13. Ellis RF, Hing WA. Neural mobilization: a systematic review of randomized controlled trials with an analysis of therapeutic efficacy. J Man Manip Ther [Internet]. 2008;16(1):8–22. Available from: http://www.ncbi.nlm.nih.gov/pubmed/19119380.
14. Rodrigues da Silva Barros B, Dal'Ava Augusto D, de Medeiros Neto JF, Michener LA, Silva RS, Sousa CDO. Isometric versus isotonic exercise in individuals with rotator cuff tendinopathy-effects on shoulder pain, functioning, muscle strength, and electromyographic activity: a protocol for randomized clinical trial. PLoS One [Internet]. 2023;18(11):e0293457. Available from: http://www.ncbi.nlm.nih.gov/pubmed/37956135.
15. Woodley BL, Newsham-West RJ, Baxter GD. Chronic tendinopathy: effectiveness of eccentric exercise. Br J Sports Med [Internet]. 2007;41(4):188–98; discussion 199. Available from: http://www.ncbi.nlm.nih.gov/pubmed/17062655.
16. Frizziero A, Pellizzon G, Vittadini F, Bigliardi D, Costantino C. Efficacy of core stability in non-specific chronic low back pain. J Funct Morphol Kinesiol [Internet]. 2021;6(2). Available from: http://www.ncbi.nlm.nih.gov/pubmed/33922389.
17. Elder A, Powers CM. Scapular stabilization for shoulder pain: putting the cart before the horse? Int J Sports Phys Ther [Internet]. 2025;20(2):275–82. Available from: http://www.ncbi.nlm.nih.gov/pubmed/39906061.
18. Riva D, Bianchi R, Rocca F, Mamo C. Proprioceptive training and injury prevention in a professional men's basketball team: a six-year prospective study. J Strength Cond Res [Internet]. 2016;30(2):461–75. Available from: http://www.ncbi.nlm.nih.gov/pubmed/26203850.
19. Manojlović D, Kopše EI. The effectiveness of aerobic exercise for pain management in patients with fibromyalgia. Eur J Transl Myol [Internet]. 2023;33(3). Available from: http://www.ncbi.nlm.nih.gov/pubmed/37449965.
20. Ketelhut S, Ketelhut RG. Type of exercise training and training methods. Adv Exp Med Biol [Internet]. 2020;1228:25–43. Available from: http://www.ncbi.nlm.nih.gov/pubmed/32342448.

21. Stavrinou PS, Astorino TA, Giannaki CD, Aphamis G, Bogdanis GC. Customizing intense interval exercise training prescription using the "frequency, intensity, time, and type of exercise" (FITT) principle. Front Physiol [Internet]. 2025;16:1553846. Available from: http://www.ncbi.nlm.nih.gov/pubmed/40247924.
22. Warden SJ, Edwards WB, Willy RW. Preventing bone stress injuries in runners with optimal workload. Curr Osteoporos Rep [Internet]. 2021;19(3):298–307. Available from: http://www.ncbi.nlm.nih.gov/pubmed/33635519.
23. Rooney D, Gilmartin E, Heron N. Prescribing exercise and physical activity to treat and manage health conditions. Ulster Med J [Internet]. 2023;92(1):9–15. Available from: http://www.ncbi.nlm.nih.gov/pubmed/36762135.
24. Morán-Navarro R, Pérez CE, Mora-Rodríguez R, de la Cruz-Sánchez E, González-Badillo JJ, Sánchez-Medina L, et al. Time course of recovery following resistance training leading or not to failure. Eur J Appl Physiol [Internet]. 2017;117(12):2387–99. Available from: http://www.ncbi.nlm.nih.gov/pubmed/28965198.
25. Ramamoorthy S, Cidlowski JA. Corticosteroids: mechanisms of action in health and disease. Rheum Dis Clin North Am [Internet]. 2016;42(1):15–31, vii. Available from: http://www.ncbi.nlm.nih.gov/pubmed/26611548.
26. Foster ZJ, Voss TT, Hatch J, Frimodig A. Corticosteroid injections for common musculoskeletal conditions. Am Fam Physician [Internet]. 2015;92(8):694–9. Available from: http://www.ncbi.nlm.nih.gov/pubmed/26554409.
27. Afridi A, Ahmad B, Ahmed H. Outcomes of single corticosteroid injection in De Quervain's tenosynovitis. Cureus [Internet]. 2024;16(10):e71928. Available from: http://www.ncbi.nlm.nih.gov/pubmed/39564036.
28. Si-Hyeong Park S, Li B, Kim C. Efficacy of intra-articular injections for the treatment of osteoarthritis: a narrative review. Osteoarthr Cartil Open [Internet]. 2025;7(2):100596. Available from: http://www.ncbi.nlm.nih.gov/pubmed/40144957.
29. Hammi C, Schroeder JD, Yeung B. Trigger point injection [internet]. StatPearls; 2026. Available from: http://www.ncbi.nlm.nih.gov/pubmed/17321283.
30. Daniels EW, Cole D, Jacobs B, Phillips SF. Existing evidence on ultrasound-guided injections in sports medicine. Orthop J Sport Med [Internet]. 2018;6(2):2325967118756576. Available from: http://www.ncbi.nlm.nih.gov/pubmed/29511701.
31. Shen P-C, Lin T-Y, Wu W-T, Özçakar L, Chang K-V. Comparison of ultrasound- vs. landmark-guided injections for musculoskeletal pain: an umbrella review. J Rehabil Med [Internet]. 2024;56:jrm40679. Available from: http://www.ncbi.nlm.nih.gov/pubmed/39185547.
32. Ruiz Santiago F, Orellana González C, Moraleda Cabrera B, Láinez Ramos-Bossini AJ. Ultrasound guided procedures in the musculoskeletal system: a narrative review with illustrative examples. Quant Imaging Med Surg [Internet]. 2024;14(11):8028–49. Available from: http://www.ncbi.nlm.nih.gov/pubmed/39544472.
33. Kamel SI, Rosas HG, Gorbachova T. Local and systemic side effects of corticosteroid injections for musculoskeletal indications. AJR Am J Roentgenol [Internet]. 2024;222(3):e2330458. Available from: http://www.ncbi.nlm.nih.gov/pubmed/38117096.
34. Stephens MB, Beutler AI, O'Connor FG. Musculoskeletal injections: a review of the evidence. Am Fam Physician [Internet]. 2008;78(8):971–6. Available from: http://www.ncbi.nlm.nih.gov/pubmed/18953975.
35. Puzzitiello RN, Patel BH, Forlenza EM, Nwachukwu BU, Allen AA, Forsythe B, et al. Adverse impact of corticosteroids on rotator cuff tendon health and repair: a systematic review of basic science studies. Arthrosc Sport Med Rehabil [Internet]. 2020;2(2). Available from: https://arthroscopyjournals.onlinelibrary.wiley.com/doi/10.1016/j.asmr.2020.01.002.
36. Chung M-W, Hsu C-Y, Chung W-K, Lin Y-N. Effects of dextrose prolotherapy on tendinopathy, fasciopathy, and ligament injuries, fact or myth?: a systematic review and meta-analysis. Medicine (Baltimore) [Internet]. 2020;99(46):e23201. Available from: http://www.ncbi.nlm.nih.gov/pubmed/33181700.
37. Conrozier T, Raman R, Diraçoglu D, Montfort J, Bard H, Baron D, et al. EUROVISCO consensus guidelines for the use of hyaluronic acid viscosupplementation in knee osteoarthritis

based on patient characteristics. Cartilage [Internet]. 2025;16(4):438–52. Available from: http://www.ncbi.nlm.nih.gov/pubmed/39564753.

38. Barreto ESR, Antunes Júnior CR, Alencar VB, Leandro MP, Leite LMB, Lins-Kusterer LEF, et al. The efficacy of botulinum toxin in tennis elbow: a meta-analysis of randomized clinical trials. Int Orthop [Internet]. 2024;48(12):3139–49. Available from: http://www.ncbi.nlm.nih.gov/pubmed/39347988.
39. Sizer PS, Brismée J-M, Cook C. Medical screening for red flags in the diagnosis and management of musculoskeletal spine pain. Pain Pract [Internet]. 2007;7(1):53–71. Available from: http://www.ncbi.nlm.nih.gov/pubmed/17305681.
40. Rao S, Riskowski JL, Hannan MT. Musculoskeletal conditions of the foot and ankle: assessments and treatment options. Best Pract Res Clin Rheumatol [Internet]. 2012;26(3):345–68. Available from: http://www.ncbi.nlm.nih.gov/pubmed/22867931.
41. Vincent HK, Heywood K, Connelly J, Hurley RW. Obesity and weight loss in the treatment and prevention of osteoarthritis. PM R [Internet]. 2012;4(5 Suppl):S59–67. Available from: http://www.ncbi.nlm.nih.gov/pubmed/22632704.
42. Hoenig T, Eissele J, Strahl A, Popp KL, Stürznickel J, Ackerman KE, et al. Return to sport following low-risk and high-risk bone stress injuries: a systematic review and meta-analysis. Br J Sports Med [Internet]. 2023;bjsports-2022-106328. Available from: https://bjsm.bmj.com/lookup/doi/10.1136/bjsports-2022-106328.
43. De la Corte-Rodriguez H, Roman-Belmonte JM, Resino-Luis C, Madrid-Gonzalez J, Rodriguez-Merchan EC. The role of physical exercise in chronic musculoskeletal pain: best medicine-a narrative review. Healthc (Basel, Switzerland) [Internet]. 2024;12(2). Available from: http://www.ncbi.nlm.nih.gov/pubmed/38255129.
44. Holm-Jensen A, Vlachos E, Storm LK, Myburgh C. Secondary prevention of musculoskeletal sports injuries: a scoping review of early detection and early intervention strategies. J Can Chiropr Assoc [Internet]. 2025;69(2):107–19. Available from: http://www.ncbi.nlm.nih.gov/pubmed/41098638.
45. Belton J, Birkinshaw H, Pincus T. Patient-centered consultations for persons with musculoskeletal conditions. Chiropr Man Therap [Internet]. 2022;30(1):53. Available from: http://www.ncbi.nlm.nih.gov/pubmed/36494862.
46. Grenfell J, Soundy A. People's experience of shared decision making in musculoskeletal physiotherapy: a systematic review and thematic synthesis. Behav Sci (Basel, Switzerland) [Internet]. 2022;12(1). Available from: http://www.ncbi.nlm.nih.gov/pubmed/35049623.
47. Menzel NN. Psychosocial factors in musculoskeletal disorders. Crit Care Nurs Clin North Am [Internet]. 2007;19(2):145–53. Available from: http://www.ncbi.nlm.nih.gov/pubmed/17512470.
48. Miller J, West J, Khawar H, Middleton R. Cauda equina syndrome. Br J Hosp Med (Lond) [Internet]. 2023;84(11):1–7. Available from: http://www.ncbi.nlm.nih.gov/pubmed/38186331.
49. Bukhary HA, Basha NA, Dobel AA, Alsufyani RM, Alotaibi RA, Almadani SH. Prevalence and pattern of injuries across the weight-training sports. Cureus [Internet]. 2023;15(11):e49759. Available from: http://www.ncbi.nlm.nih.gov/pubmed/38046743.

The manufacturer's authorised representative in the EU is Springer Nature Customer Service Centre GmbH, Europaplatz 3, 69115 Heidelberg, Germany. If you have any concerns regarding our products, please contact ProductSafety@springernature.com

Printed and bound by CPI Group (UK) Ltd, Croydon, CR0 4YY
23/10/2026
02238453-0001